Dyspepsia
Dyspepsia

Emad M El-Omar BSc (Hons), MB ChB (Glas),
FRCP (Edin), MD
*Professor of Gastroenterology and Honorary
Consultant Physician*
Aberdeen University and Aberdeen Royal Infirmary,
Aberdeen, UK

Richard M Peek Jr MD
*Associate Professor of Gastroenterology and Cancer
Biology*
Division of Gastroenterology, Vanderbilt University
School of Medicine, Nashville, Tennessee, USA

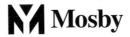 Mosby

85

Acknowledgements

We are both very grateful to our friends and colleagues for their valuable comments and advice about all aspects of this book.

MOSBY
An imprint of Elsevier Limited.

© 2003 Elsevier Limited.

The
Publisher's
policy is to use
**paper manufactured
from sustainable forests**

M **Mosby** is a registered trademark of Elsevier Limited.

ISBN 0-7234-3326-7

Cataloguing in Publication Data
Catalogue records for this book are available from the US Library of Congress and the British Library.

Note
Medical knowledge is constantly changing. As new information becomes available, changes in treatment, procedures, equipment and the use of drugs become neces-sary. The editors/authors/contributors and the publishers have taken care to ensure that the information given in this text is accurate and up to date. However, readers are strongly advised to confirm that the information, especially with regard to drug usage, complies with the latest legislation and standards of practice. Website address-es correct at time of going to press.

Printed by Grafos S.A. Arte sobre papel, Spain.

4/29/04

Contents

Foreword

Dyspepsia is probably the commonest, chronic disorder affecting humans. It impairs quality of life and may be associated with potentially serious underlying disease.

Over the past few years, there have been marked advances in our understanding of the aetiology of dyspeptic disease, the most marked being the recognition of the role of *Helicobacter pylori* infection in peptic ulcer disease. There have also been changes in the recommendations regarding appropriate investigations in younger patients with uncomplicated dyspepsia with non-invasive *H. pylori* testing replacing routine endoscopy. Even the definition of dyspepsia has changed over the past few years. For all these reasons, this rapid reference on dyspepsia is both timely and welcomed.

Professor El-Omar and Dr Peek are widely respected and admired for their clinical experience and expertise in dyspeptic disease and for their internationally recognised research work into these disorders. They are ideally qualified to produce a clinically relevant and academically sound review of this area. Their review of the subject is both comprehensive and concise.

I am sure this publication will be of immense value to a wide range of readers. This includes clinicians in both primary and secondary care, as well as those who have an interest in the underlying mechanisms of dyspeptic disease.

Professor Kenneth E.L. McColl, Western Infirmary, Glasgow, UK

Abbreviations

C-RP	C-reactive protein
DGM	duodenal gastric metaplasia
ESR	erythrocyte sedimentation rate
FD	functional dyspepsia
FOB	faecal occult blood
GI	gastrointestinal
GORD	gastro-oesophageal reflux disease
IBD	inflammatory bowel disease
IBS	irritable bowel syndrome
LOS	lower oesophageal sphincter
NERD	non-erosive reflux disease
NSAID	non-steroidal anti-inflammatory drug
NUD	non-ulcer dyspepsia
PPI	proton pump inhibitor
PUD	peptic ulcer disease
RUT	rapid urease test
SSRI	selective serotonin reuptake inhibitors
UBT	urea breath test

Introduction and Background

The word dyspepsia, also known as "indigestion" to the lay public, is a Latin word derived from the Greek words *dys* (bad) and *pepsis* (digestion). Most people regard it as a manifestation of malfunction of the digestive system, but in reality it comprises a group of symptoms that point towards disease of the upper gastrointestinal (GI) tract. This relationship to the upper GI tract, and to eating in particular, has long been recognized and prompted a 19th century writer to describe dyspepsia as "*the remorse of a guilty stomach*". The other important feature of dyspepsia is its persistent or recurrent nature; in other words, it is a chronic condition. Dyspepsia represents a major health problem in most societies and billions of pounds are spent annually on its investigation and treatment. In this book, we hope to give an overview of its definition, aetiology, clinical manifestations and treatment. We do acknowledge, however, that such a topic is bound to generate differences of opinion and heated discussions but we strive to negotiate a middle road guided by the accepted balance of evidence available in the literature.

Definitions of Dyspepsia

What is dyspepsia?

Dyspepsia is difficult to define as it is not a diagnosis, but rather a collection of symptoms. The simplest definition is pain or discomfort in the upper abdomen. However, the spectrum of symptoms that is encompassed by "dyspepsia" includes upper abdominal discomfort, retrosternal pain, anorexia, nausea, vomiting, bloating, fullness, early satiety and heartburn.[1,2] The terms "**investigated**" and "**uninvestigated**" dyspepsia are often used in relation to patients in whom diagnostic investigations had or had not been undertaken in the evaluation of their dyspeptic symptoms. Dyspeptic symptoms are poor discriminators of clinical diagnoses as many diseases cause dyspepsia, including peptic ulcers, oesophagitis, gastric or pancreatic neoplasia and cholelithiasis. Dyspepsia that is caused by an organic condition such as the ones mentioned above is known as "**organic dyspepsia**". In approximately 50% of cases, no clear pathological cause for a patient's symptoms can be determined and the term "**functional**" or "**non-ulcer dyspepsia (NUD)**" is used (Figure 1). These terms are interchangeable to some extent and imply that essential investigations such as upper GI endoscopy and abdominal ultrasound have excluded gastroduodenal and hepatobiliary abnormalities. Clearly the terms organic and functional dyspepsia can only be ascribed to investigated patients, while uninvestigated patients may simply be prescribed empirical treatment without ever finding out the aetiology of their complaint.

Formal definitions of dyspepsia

ROME I

There have been several consensus definitions of dyspepsia developed by international working parties. Perhaps the most widely known is the 1991 ROME I definition, which defines dyspepsia as "persistent or recurrent abdominal pain or abdominal discomfort centred in the upper abdomen and considered to be

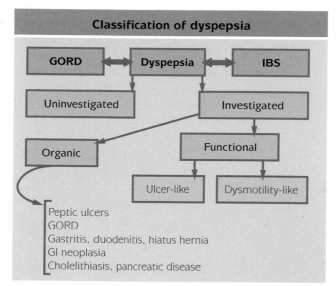

Figure 1. Classification of dyspepsia.

related to the upper alimentary tract".[3] Discomfort may be characterized by postprandial fullness, early satiety, nausea, retching, vomiting and upper abdominal bloating (sensation of distension as distinct from visible distension). Duration is not specified in the definition as patients may present immediately following onset (Table 1). The pain or discomfort may or may not be related to meals and may be intermittent or continuous.

Symptom subgroups in dyspepsia

For convenience purposes, the ROME I criteria classified dyspeptic symptoms into subgroups termed ulcer-like, reflux-like and dysmotility-like. Although this may imply some correlation with actual pathological findings, these symptom subgroups correlate very poorly with pathophysiological abnormalities.[4] Furthermore, there is a large degree of overlap between the symptom subgroups.[5–7] For example, many peptic ulcer patients complain of reflux-like or dysmotility-like symptoms while having classic ulcer-like symptoms. The following section describes the most widely known symptom subgroups.

The spectrum of dyspepsia symptoms and recommended definitions

Symptom	Definition
Pain centred in the upper abdomen	Pain refers to a subjective, unpleasant sensation; some patients may feel that tissue damage is occurring. Other symptoms may be extremely bothersome without being interpreted by the patient as pain. By questioning the patient, pain should be distinguished from discomfort.
Discomfort centred in the upper abdomen	A subjective, unpleasant sensation or feeling that is not interpreted as pain according to the patient and which, if fully assessed, can include any of the symptoms below.
Early satiety	A feeling that the stomach is overfilled soon after starting to eat, out of proportion to the size of the meal being eaten, so that the meal cannot be finished.
Fullness	An unpleasant sensation like the persistence of food in the stomach; this may or may not occur postprandially (slow digestion).
Bloating in the upper abdomen	A tightness located in the upper abdomen; it should be distinguished from visible abdominal distension.
Nausea	Queasiness or sick sensation; a feeling of the need to vomit.

Table 1. The spectrum of dyspepsia symptoms and recommended definitions. Reproduced with permission from Talley NJ *et al*. Functional gastroduodenal disorders. *Gut* 1999; **45**(Suppl II): II37–II42.

Ulcer-like dyspepsia
- Epigastric pain is the predominant symptom (pain below diaphragm).
- Pain is periodic and frequently nocturnal.
- Pain occurs between meals or when the stomach is empty (hunger pains).
- Pain is relieved by food, antacids or acid-inhibitory agents.

Dysmotility-like dyspepsia
- Upper abdominal discomfort is the predominant symptom and is not usually nocturnal.
- Pain is not a major feature.
- Symptoms aggravated by eating.
- Early satiety.
- Postprandial fullness.
- Bloating.
- Recurrent nausea and/or vomiting.
- Some have variable and multiple food intolerance.

Reflux-like dyspepsia
- Reflux-like dyspepsia is no longer regarded as part of the spectrum of functional dyspepsia.
- Heartburn and regurgitation.
- Pain above diaphragm.
- Substernal burning pain, which may radiate into neck or throat and usually occurs after large meals and when stooping or lying flat.
- History of recent weight gain.

ROME II
Despite their wide use in research, the ROME I criteria for gastroduodenal disorders remained contentious. The main criticism is centred on the lack of usefulness of these criteria in predicting gastroduodenal pathology. In an attempt to resolve these issues, an international panel of clinical investigators reviewed the available evidence and arrived at a consensus statement that classified functional gastroduodenal disorders

(category B) into different groups (ROME II).[8] This revised classification does not apply to patients with predominant heartburn or irritable bowel syndrome (IBS)-related dyspepsia. It is thought that heartburn and/or acid regurgitation are sufficiently accurate predictors of gastro-oesophageal reflux disease to make a reasonable diagnosis, while IBS symptoms usually involve some reference to bowel function that again makes it unlikely that the upper GI tract is involved. Thus, the new groups are defined below.

- **Functional dyspepsia (category B1):** defined as having symptoms for at least 12 weeks, which need not be consecutive, within the preceding 12 months of:
  (1) persistent or recurrent dyspepsia (pain or discomfort centred in the upper abdomen); and
  (2) no evidence of organic disease (particularly after upper GI endoscopy) that is likely to explain the symptoms; and
  (3) no evidence that dyspepsia is exclusively relieved by defecation or associated with the onset of a change in stool frequency or stool form (i.e. not irritable bowel).

- **Aerophagia (category B2):** defined as having at least 12 weeks, which need not be consecutive, in the preceding 12 months of:
  (1) air swallowing that is objectively observed; and
  (2) troublesome repetitive belching.

- **Functional vomiting (category B3):** defined as having at least 12 weeks, which need not be consecutive, in the preceding 12 months of:
  (1) frequent episodes of vomiting, occurring on at least 3 separate days in a week; and
  (2) absence of criteria for an eating disorder, rumination, or major psychiatric disease according to DSM-IV; and
  (3) absence of self-induced and medication-induced vomiting; and
  (4) absence of abnormalities in the gut or central nervous system, and metabolic diseases to explain the recurrent vomiting.

In addition, the panel proposed symptom subgroups for functional dyspepsia based on patient ranking of the most bothersome complaint. The new symptom subgroups are:

- **Ulcer-like dyspepsia (B1a):** the predominant or most bothersome symptom is **pain** centred in the upper abdomen. The features of this predominant pain are similar to the description given earlier.
- **Dysmotility-like dyspepsia (B1b):** the predominant symptom is an unpleasant or troublesome non-painful sensation **(discomfort)** centred in the upper abdomen. This sensation may be characterized by or associated with upper abdominal fullness, early satiety, bloating, or nausea, as in the old descriptions given earlier.
- **Unspecified (non-specific) dyspepsia:** this includes symptomatic patients whose symptoms do not fulfil the criteria for ulcer-like or dysmotility-like dyspepsia.

Epidemiology

Prevalence

Dyspepsia is a very common complaint with an estimated 5% of visits to primary care physicians being due to dyspepsia.[9] Penston and Pounder examined the prevalence of dyspeptic symptoms in a representative sample of the adult population (aged 16 or above) of Great Britain.[5] Of the 2112 subjects questioned, 40% reported having had one or more dyspeptic symptoms in the previous year, and about a half of them described these symptoms as being moderate to severe. Of this group, more than half were taking drugs for dyspepsia (40% of which were prescribed) and 22% had seen their general practitioner about dyspepsia in the previous year. Thus, 9% of all those interviewed reported consulting their physician about dyspepsia in the previous year. Overall, 2% of the survey sample had been absent from work due to dyspepsia. Surveys from other Western societies have recorded prevalences of between 23 and 41%.

Whether dyspepsia is becoming more common is unclear, but general practice consultations for non-ulcer dyspepsia have been increasing. Between 1981–2 and 1991–2 there was an 85% increase in the number of patients presenting with upper GI disorders in general practitioner morbidity surveys. In contrast, morbidity and mortality resulting from peptic ulcer disease fell by 9% in the same period.[10]

The prevalence of dyspepsia is slightly higher in women and declines slightly with age.[11]

Economic cost of dyspepsia

Dyspeptic diseases place a heavy economic burden on most societies. Direct costs are incurred from visits to doctors, expensive diagnostic tests and medications, while indirect costs are due to absenteeism and diminished productivity in the workplace.[12] Another important drain on resources is the cost of managing complications such as gastrointestinal bleeding or perforation from peptic ulceration and oesophagitis.

To illustrate the scale of the burden imposed by dyspeptic diseases, one need only consider the cost of endoscopy and treatment of the condition. Although only 10% of patients attending their general practitioner with dyspepsia will be referred for hospital consultation or investigation, this still represents one of the commonest reasons for referral to hospital. The number of upper GI endoscopies performed annually in the UK has risen steadily over the past decade. In 1996, over 450,000 endoscopies were performed at a cost of £80–£450 per procedure depending on the hospital.[10] This represents approximately one endoscopy for every 100 adults in England and Wales. If one also adds the figures for barium studies, 2% of the entire adult population receive either an endoscopy or barium meal each year.

In terms of treatment, up to 4% of the population are thought to be taking prescribed drugs for dyspepsia at any one time. These drugs account for over 10% of drug expenditure in primary care (£471 million in 1999 in England and Wales).[10]

Time lost from work and interference with quality of life are more difficult to measure but are likely to be considerable.

Among the drugs used to treat dyspeptic diseases, the proton pump inhibitors (PPIs) are the most expensive class of drug in the UK, costing nearly £300 million in 1998. Attempts at reducing expenditure on PPIs prompted the UK National Institute for Clinical Excellence (NICE) to issue some guidelines on appropriate prescription of these drugs.[13]

Aetiology

The definition of dyspepsia understandably allows for a large differential diagnosis. As mentioned earlier, 40–50% of dyspeptic patients have an underlying organic illness, with the rest having functional dyspepsia. Dyspeptic symptoms frequently accompany GI tract as well as systemic disorders. The following is a non-exhaustive list of the differential diagnosis of dyspepsia.

Gastrointestinal tract disorders

- Functional dyspepsia (non-ulcer dyspepsia). By far the commonest single cause, accounting for at least half the patients, especially the young.
- Peptic ulcer disease. Most patients with peptic ulcers have dyspepsia but only 15–20% of dyspeptic patients are found to have peptic ulcers.
- Gastric erythema, duodenal erythema or hiatus hernia. Frequent and may be found exclusively or in combination with other endoscopic findings.
- Gastro-oesophageal reflux disease (GORD). This may manifest endoscopically as erosive oesophagitis or non-erosive reflux diseases (NERD). GORD is very frequent and increasing in incidence. There is a large overlap between symptoms of dyspepsia and those of GORD. Approximately 15% of dyspeptic patients have endoscopic evidence of oesophagitis (with or without heartburn).
- Gastric or oesophageal malignancy. Found in approximately 2% of patients, 98% of whom are older than 45 years of age.
- Gastroparesis. Caused by metabolic or endocrine abnormalities such as diabetic autonomic neuropathy, hyper- or hypothyroidism, adrenal insufficiency and hypercalcaemia. Gastroparesis could also be due to neuropathic conditions such as Parkinson's disease or Shy–Drager syndrome, or commonly following a viral infection.
- Mesenteric vascular insufficiency characterized by postprandial pain, weight loss and a fear of eating.

- Other rare causes: Crohn's disease, lymphocytic and oeosinophilic gastritis, Ménétrier's syndrome, coeliac disease, ischaemic bowel disease, carbohydrate malabsorption (e.g. lactose, fructose or sorbitol intolerance), parasitic infections (e.g. *Giardia lamblia* is very common in developing countries; strongyloides).

Medications

Many drugs have significant GI side effects and several have a propensity to cause dyspeptic symptoms. This may be due to direct irritation of the gastric mucosa, alteration of gastric motility, relaxation of lower oesophageal sphincter thus provoking reflux, co-ingestion of substances used in the formulation of the drugs such as sorbitol or lactose, or unknown mechanisms. The best known drugs associated with dyspeptic symptoms are listed below.

Drugs that are most likely to cause dyspepsia
- Non-steroidal anti-inflammatory drugs (NSAIDs)
- Digoxin
- Antibiotics (macrolides, metronidazole)
- Corticosteroids, oestrogens
- Iron, potassium chloride
- Levodopa
- Theophylline
- Quinidine
- Niacin, gemfibrozil
- Colchicine

Drugs associated with dyspepsia
- Alendronic acid
- Aspirin
- Azithromycin
- Carbergoline
- Clopidogrel
- Gabapentin
- Indapamide
- Itraconazole

- Mycophenolate
- Nedocromil
- NSAIDs (all types)
- Pergolide
- Potassium supplements
- Risperidone
- Ritonavir
- Rivastigmine
- Sildenafil
- SSRIs
- Stanozolol
- Tacrolimus
- Theophylline
- Tolterodine
- Zidovudine

Drugs associated with gastro-oesophageal reflux
- Anticholinergics
- Beta 2 agonists
- Calcium channel blockers
- Hormones
- Nitrates
- NSAIDs
- Oral contraceptives
- Smooth muscle relaxants
- Theophylline

Pancreaticobiliary disorders
- Cholelithiasis or choledocholithiasis: many patients have asymptomatic cholelithiasis but a substantial proportion will present with dyspeptic symptoms.
- Acute or chronic relapsing pancreatitis characterized by episodic dull steady upper abdominal pain that may be aggravated by meals and radiate through to the back.
- Pancreatic malignancy.

Systemic disorders

- Diabetes mellitus: poor glycaemic control is frequently associated with dyspepsia, and serious complications such as diabetic ketoacidosis present with nausea and vomiting in most patients. Diabetic gastroparesis is also frequently associated with dyspeptic symptoms.
- Hypo- or hyperthyroidism.
- Hyperparathyroidism: the associated hypercalcaemia is a recognized cause of peptic ulcer disease.
- Ischaemic heart disease: acute myocardial infarction occasionally presents as an epigastric pain or discomfort, and some patients merely present with nausea and vomiting.
- Connective tissue disorders: e.g. scleroderma and systemic lupus erythematosus.
- Chronic renal failure: especially patients on dialysis.
- Pregnancy: apart from nausea and vomiting of early pregnancy, a significant percentage of women complain of reflux and dysmotility-like symptoms during advanced pregnancy.

Clinical Features of Dyspepsia

Many studies have shown that establishing a diagnosis from individual GI symptoms alone is difficult. Even in clear cut organic entities such as duodenal ulcer, the clinician is right in less than 50% of cases, i.e. worse than tossing a coin! Obviously different diseases do have a different spectrum of symptoms. Thus patients with gastric cancer frequently complain of profound anorexia, weight loss and nausea, while those with alcohol related dyspepsia typically vomit and retch, especially early in the morning. Other differences that stand out include the frequent use of psychotropic drugs in functional dyspepsia and the high incidence of heartburn in oesophageal disease.

However, even seemingly serious indicators such as substantial weight loss (>3 kg), anorexia and nausea are surprisingly common in functional dyspepsia, which, being so much commoner than gastric cancer, accounts for far more cases. Thus, most symptoms are neither specific nor sensitive for any particular condition. Even the classic features of peptic ulcer such as relief of pain by antacids or food and nocturnal pain, though commoner in peptic ulcer (65%, 75%, and 75% respectively), are sufficiently common in functional dyspepsia (60%, 40%, and 43% respectively) to be unhelpful in differential diagnosis.

One exception perhaps is biliary colic. This typically is located in the right upper quadrant and radiates to the tip of the shoulder and occurs in attacks with long periods of freedom from pain. If pain develops in the late evening, lasts over 2 hours, and is associated with sweating and vomiting, then biliary colic is likely.

Table 2 lists the frequency of certain gastrointestinal symptoms in certain dyspepsia related diseases and in a later chapter of this book the clinical features of organic dyspepsias will be discussed in more detail.

Gastrointestinal symptoms in dyspepsia related diseases								
Symptom	**% of patients with specified symptom**							
	FD	**OES**	**DU**	**GU**	**IBS**	**GS**	**ARD**	**GC**
Anorexia	40	35	47	56	35	29	55	64*
Nausea	39	17	34	39	32	28	37	48*
Vomiting	24	22	34	34	11*	23	59*	49
GI bleed	12	14	26*	23	5	7	32	34*
Heartburn	20	64*	32	23	12	19	25	22
Weight loss	23	20	26	34	16*	32	33	72
Psychotropic drug use	46*	35	26	20	38	31	18	9*

FD = functional dyspepsia; OES = oesophagitis and reflux without oesophagitis; DU = duodenal ulcer; GU = gastric ulcer; IBS = irritable bowel syndrome; GS = gallstone disease; ARD = alcohol related dyspepsia; GC = gastric cancer.
*Significant difference from other diseases.

Table 2. Gastrointestinal symptoms in dyspepsia related diseases. Reproduced with permission from Spiller RC. ABC of the upper gastrointestinal tract: Anorexia, nausea, vomiting and pain *BMJ* 2001; **323:**1354–1357.

Alarm symptoms/signs in dyspepsia

The presence of the following symptoms or signs should always be taken seriously by the primary care physician and appropriate referral to a specialist unit should be made. This is particularly important in patients who are older than 55 years of age.

- Weight loss
- Anorexia
- Dysphagia
- Odynophagia
- Persistent vomiting
- Anaemia
- Jaundice
- Evidence of GI bleeding (e.g. haematemesis, melaena, faecal occult blood (FOB) positive stool)
- Abdominal mass on examination
- Epigastric pain severe enough to hospitalize the patient
- Use of NSAIDs

- Previous gastric surgery
- Suspicious barium meal
- Family history of gastric cancer

Tools for measuring dyspepsia

There have been several attempts at designing a questionnaire-based tool for measuring dyspepsia. Some use a simple Likert scale to assess specific symptoms while others are more detailed and robust. Two examples of the latter category have been published and gained wide acceptance: the Nepean Dyspepsia Index,[14] which was designed in Australia and measures the multi-dimensional impact of dyspepsia, and the Glasgow Dyspepsia Severity Score (GDSS),[15] which was designed by our group in Scotland. The GDSS questionnaire (Figure 2) records frequency of symptoms, effect on routine activities, time off work, frequency of medical consultations, clinical investigations and use of over-the-counter and prescribed medications. This tool was found to be highly reproducible and has high validity and responsiveness. In addition, it is simple and rapid to perform. It provides a valuable tool for assessing the response to treatment in patients with dyspepsia. The tool is flexible and could be adjusted to measure dyspeptic symptoms over 1 year, 6 months, 3 months, or even 6 weeks. We found it extremely useful in the assessment of dyspeptic symptoms before and after *Helicobacter pylori* eradication therapy in patients with functional dyspepsia and peptic ulcer disease.[16–18]

Physical examination

Examination of most dyspeptic patients will be normal but one should look out for particular signs that suggest significant pathology (Figure 3). Some patients will have tenderness to palpation, but this is a very poor discriminating sign and is frequently found in patients with functional dyspepsia. Signs of anaemia indicate chronic blood loss, perhaps from an ulcer. Presence of an abdominal mass is ominous and is an indication for urgent investigations. A sucussion splash suggests obstruction of the gastric outlet and abdominal distension and hyperactive bowel sounds may indicate small bowel obstruction. FOB testing is mandatory for all dyspeptic patients.

The Glasgow Dyspepsia Severity Score (GDSS)

(A) Over the past 6 months, have you experienced upper abdominal and/or chest discomfort?

0 = Never
1 = On only 1 or 2 days
2 = On approx. 1 day per month
3 = On approx. 1 day per week
4 = On approx. 50% of days
5 = On most days

(B) When you are experiencing the discomfort, is it usually:

1 = Mild, i.e. aware of it but does not interfere with normal activities, or
2 = Moderate, i.e. tolerable but does interfere with normal activities, or
3 = Severe, i.e. intolerable and prevents normal activities e.g. time off work etc.?

(C) How many days have you lost off work due to your dyspepsia in the last 6 months?

0 = None
1 = 1–7
2 = More than 7 days

(D) How often have you seen a doctor due to dyspepsia in the past 6 months?

0 = None
1 = Once
2 = Twice or more

(E) How often have you called your GP to visit you at home in the past 6 months?

0 = None
1 = Once
2 = Twice or more

(F) Give details of any tests you have had for your dyspepsia in the past 6 months

0 = None
1 = One
2 = Two or more tests

Continued...

Figure 2. The Glasgow Dyspepsia Severity Score (GDSS).

The Glasgow Dyspepsia Severity Score (GDSS) *Continued*

(G) Details of treatment taken for dyspepsia over the past 6 months

(1) Over the last 6 months, how frequently have you used drugs available over the counter?

0 = None
1 = Less than once per week
2 = More than once per week

Name of Drug

1. .... 2. ....
3. .... 4. ....

(2) Over the last 6 months, for how long have you used drugs only obtainable on prescription?

0 = None
1 = For 1 month or less
2 = For 1–3 months
3 = For more than 3 months

Name of Drug

1. .... 2. ....
3. .... 4. ....

TOTAL GDSS SCORE =

Physical examination of dyspeptic patients

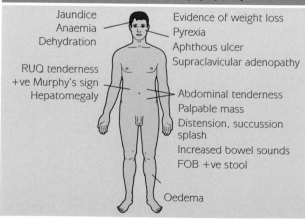

Jaundice
Anaemia
Dehydration

RUQ tenderness
+ve Murphy's sign
Hepatomegaly

Evidence of weight loss
Pyrexia
Aphthous ulcer
Supraclavicular adenopathy

Abdominal tenderness
Palpable mass
Distension, succussion splash
Increased bowel sounds
FOB +ve stool

Oedema

Figure 3. Physical examination of dyspeptic patients. FOB, faecal occult blood; RUQ, right upper quadrant.

Investigations of Dyspepsia

The decision to investigate dyspepsia is clearly dependent on the severity and duration of the symptoms, the presence of alarm symptoms or signs and the availability of specialist diagnostic services within the catchment area. Although the majority of the population experience dyspeptic symptoms at some stage, only half will ever seek medical advice and this usually occurs within 6 months of the onset of these symptoms.[19] Understandably, the primary care physician's main responsibility is to ensure that no significant pathology is being missed. In the absence of alarming or chronic symptoms, the general practitioner (GP) is often able to either prescribe an empirical therapy such as an acid inhibitor, or to adopt a test and treat policy for *H. pylori* infection (as will be discussed later). Thus, only a minority of dyspeptic patients ever get investigated (approximately 10%). In patients with a worrying presentation or in those where empirical therapy has failed, the GP is obliged to make the referral to a specialist for further investigations. In the context of dyspepsia, the most useful investigation is upper GI endoscopy.

Who should undergo upper GI endoscopy

Age and symptoms

The fear of missing a gastric malignancy has long dictated policy regarding the use of upper GI endoscopy to investigate dyspepsia. However, the incidence of gastric cancer is age-dependent and very few cases present below the age of 55.[20] Even then, the presentation of gastric cancer in younger patients is usually alarming enough to prompt invasive investigations in any case. Provided alarm symptoms and/or signs are excluded, there is no evidence that curable gastric cancer would be missed by instituting initial empiric treatment, without resort to endoscopy, in dyspeptic patients younger than 55 years of age.[20–22] It is generally recommended that patients over the age of 55 with new onset of uncomplicated dyspepsia should be investigated with endoscopy, although this recommendation may change in the next few years.

When should the GP refer a dyspeptic patient to a specialist?

- Presence of alarm symptoms necessitating prompt investigation.
- Severe or distressing pain.
- Failure of symptoms to resolve or substantially improve after appropriate treatment, whether empirical or specific.
- Progressive symptoms.

Upper GI endoscopy (Figure 4)

Endoscopy will yield a specific diagnosis in 50–75% of cases. Although the procedure is relatively simple and safe, it is not totally risk-free. Death from diagnostic endoscopy is reported in the range of 1 in 2000–10,000, though these figures also include in-patients who may have serious co-morbid disease. In out-patient practice the rate is likely to be even lower, but any death is unacceptable. Sedation could be given if required,

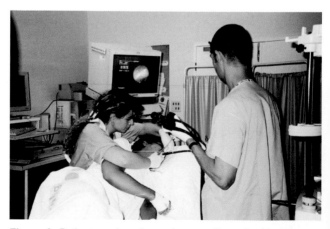

Figure 4. Patients undergoing endoscopy. Reproduced with permission from Aspinall R, Taylor-Robinson S. *Mosby's Color Atlas and Text of Gastroenterology and Liver Disease*. London: Mosby, 2001; p. 12.

although up to 50% of patients prefer to have no sedation at all. The most commonly used sedatives are the benzodiazepines, diazemuls and midazolam. Endoscopy allows the gastro-enterologist to check for *H. pylori* infection using the rapid urease slide test (most commonly used brand is the CLO test). As will be discussed later, testing for *H. pylori* infection is perhaps the most useful diagnostic test after endoscopy, and many would argue is the only test required in the absence of alarm symptoms.

Testing for evidence of *H. pylori* infection

This will be discussed in detail later but suffice to say here that this could be achieved by invasive and non-invasive means. The gold standard is actually a non-invasive method that utilizes the ^{13}C- or ^{14}C-urea breath test. Serological testing is also useful, particularly if provided as a validated laboratory-based service as opposed to a commercially available kit.

Radiological imaging

If symptoms occur in discrete attacks then ultrasound investigation of the gall bladder should be considered to exclude cholelithiasis. If malignancy is suspected outside the upper GI tract, then computed tomography of the abdomen/chest is useful. Although double contrast barium radiology is very accurate at detecting upper GI abnormalities (indeed this forms the basis of mass screening for gastric cancer in Japan), it does not allow for biopsies to be taken and is thus considered inferior to endoscopy. However, it is very useful in certain circumstances such as assessing the anatomy of the upper GI tract (e.g. strictures), motility disorders and gastro-oesophageal reflux, extrinsic and intra-mural abnormalities, and the diagnosis of malrotations, herniations and other structural abnormalities.

Ambulatory 24-hour pH monitoring and oesophageal manometry

This is discussed under gastro-oesophageal reflux disease (page 51).

Organic Causes of Dyspepsia

In this section we will discuss specific organic causes of dyspepsia. These will include peptic ulcers, gastric cancer, oesophagitis, gastritis, duodenitis and cholelithiasis.

Peptic ulcers

Peptic ulcer disease (PUD) used to be extremely common but its incidence has gradually declined in the past 2–3 decades. The incidence and prevalence show considerable geographic variation even within the same country. The life-time prevalence of PUD is approximately 10%. The incidence has dramatically fallen in the younger population with a less marked fall in those of middle and older ages. In subjects older than 65 years, the incidence of PUD has continued to rise. The fall in PUD incidence has been more marked for duodenal ulcers than for gastric ulcers. Munnangi and Sonnenberg reported on the time trends of visits to physicians for PUD.[23] Four million people visited their physician for PUD in 1995, representing a rate of 1500 per 100,000 of the US population. There has been a marked decline in physician visits for duodenal ulcer between 1958 and 1995, but visits for gastric ulcer remained unchanged.

Since the discovery of *H. pylori* infection and the widespread implementation of eradication therapy in infected ulcer patients, there has been a dramatic change in presentation of peptic ulcers, their complications and long-term management. The most obvious change is the virtual disappearance of the surgical approach to benign non-complicated peptic ulcers. Only in the extreme situations of gastric outlet obstruction, perforation or uncontrollable acute bleeding is surgery considered.

The causes and associations of peptic ulcers are varied and fascinating. Table 3 lists most of the recognized aetiologies of PUD. The main culprits are *H. pylori* infection, NSAIDs and stress ulceration in the context of severe metabolic or physical trauma. We will discuss the main clinical entities under the spectrum of PUD, namely gastritis, duodenitis, duodenal and

Aetiology of peptic ulcer disease	
Common causes of PUD	*H. pylori* infection NSAID use Stress

Uncommon causes of PUD	Gastrinoma (Zollinger–Ellison syndrome)
	Crohn's disease
	Antral G-cell hyperplasia
	Other infections
	  (e.g. cytomegalovirus, herpes simplex
	  type 1, tuberculosis)
	Chronic renal failure
	Cirrhosis of the liver
	Hypercalcaemia
	  (e.g. hyperparathyroidism)
	Enteric ischaemia
	Radiation
	Tumour spread from adjacent organs
	  (e.g. pancreas, sarcoma)

Table 3. Aetiology of peptic ulcer disease.

gastric ulcers, NSAID ulcers and stress ulcers. *H. pylori* itself
will be discussed in great detail later in the book.

Duodenal ulcers (Figure 5)

Clinical features

It is wrong to give the impression that history or clinical
examination can accurately identify PUD, or distinguish
between duodenal and gastric ulcers. Unfortunately, classic
duodenal ulcer symptoms (such as hunger and nocturnal pain)
often occur in patients with functional dyspepsia, and many
patients with an ulcer have atypical complaints or are
completely asymptomatic. Misiewicz concluded that, in the
absence of endoscopic evidence, the presence or absence of
symptoms cannot be assumed to indicate with certainty the
presence or the absence of a peptic ulcer.[24]

There is a strong familial component with 20% of first-
degree relatives being affected. This may reflect intra-familial

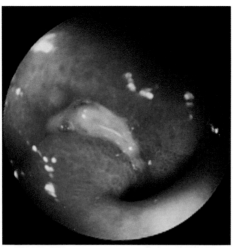

Figure 5.
Duodenal ulcer. Reproduced with permission from Silverstein FE, Tytgat GNJ. *Gastrointestinal Endoscopy*, 3rd Edition. London: Mosby, 1997; p. 220.

aggregation of *H. pylori* infection but there is also the possibility of a specific genetic factor, perhaps related to parietal cell mass or sensitivity to gastrin. Environmental factors are also implicated, with smoking and stressful life style being the most commonly cited. Studies have shown that while these do not actually cause ulceration, they are known to increase acid secretion and retard healing of established ulcers. However, such studies were conducted in the pre-*H. pylori* era and it is not clear how relevant they are today. Table 4 lists the most classical duodenal ulcer clinical features.

Pathogenesis
Pathogenesis will be discussed under *H. pylori* infection.

Investigations
Endoscopy
This remains the test of choice to rule out peptic ulceration, but its presence can now be inferred by indirect testing for *H. pylori* infection. In the absence of alarm symptoms, *H. pylori* causes 90% of duodenal ulcers and 70% of gastric ulcers; aspirin and NSAIDs account for most of the remainder. Patients who are not infected with *H. pylori* and not taking NSAIDs

Clinical features of duodenal ulcer disease
• Younger patients (particularly men) are most often affected.
• Strong familial component: 20% of first-degree relatives are affected.
• Main symptom is epigastric pain, which classically occurs when the stomach is empty: "hunger pain" and "nocturnal pain".
• The patients points to the epigastrium when asked to locate the pain: "the pointing sign".
• The disease has a remitting and relapsing nature with periods of exacerbations lasting for weeks at a time.
• Vomiting and weight loss are unusual.
• Epigastric tenderness is frequently the only finding on clinical examination, unless complications such as pyloric stenosis are present.

Table 4. Clinical features of duodenal ulcer disease.

have a very low probability of ulcer disease. In the case of a straightforward chronic duodenal ulcer, the only biopsies needed are those to diagnose *H. pylori* infection (e.g. urease slide test). However, if multiple ulcers are encountered and especially if these extend into the second part of duodenum (post-bulbar ulcers), it is important to take biopsies to exclude uncommon conditions (listed in Table 5).

Causes of post-bulbar ulcers
Crohn's disease
Zollinger–Ellison syndrome (check fasting gastrin level)
Lymphoma
Carcinoma
Ectopic pancreatic tissue
Tuberculosis

Table 5. Causes of post-bulbar ulcers.

Causes of *H. pylori*-negative duodenal ulcers
False-negative test (e.g. due to concurrent PPI therapy, recent antibiotic or bismuth therapy, or insensitive method of detection)
Covert NSAID use
Crohn's disease
Zollinger–Ellison syndrome
Gastric acid hypersecretion and increased duodenal acid load
Penetrating carcinoma of the pancreas, or lymphoma

Table 6. Causes of *H. pylori*-negative duodenal ulcers.

The problem of H. pylori-negative duodenal ulcers

The overwhelming majority of duodenal ulcers are caused by *H. pylori* infection. However, there is an increasing recognition that *H. pylori*-negative ulcers (the so-called CLO negative ulcers) are becoming more common, even allowing for the increasing use of NSAIDs.[25,26] It appears that the increase in the proportion of *H. pylori*-negative duodenal ulcers is particularly prominent in areas of the world with a low or rapidly decreasing *H. pylori* prevalence. It has to be emphasized that most of the negative ulcers are caused by insensitive methods of *H. pylori* diagnosis. The cause of true *H. pylori*-negative ulceration appears to be multifactorial.[27,28] It is generally accepted that *H. pylori*-negative ulcers are more difficult to control with antisecretory drugs. Table 6 lists potential causes of a *H. pylori*-negative duodenal ulcer.

Blood tests

A routine full blood count and film is helpful to rule out anaemia. A serum ferritin would be useful to assess iron stores in cases of anaemia. A fasting plasma gastrin is useful if Zollinger–Ellison syndrome is suspected.

Complications of duodenal ulcers

Complications of duodenal ulcers (Table 7) have become less common over the past decade. This is mainly due to the recognition and treatment of *H. pylori* infection. Most of the complicated ulcers are now due to NSAID use in the elderly, particularly in

Complications of duodenal ulcers	
Complication	**Comment**
Recurrence	90% within 2 years if *H. pylori* is not eradicated; risk of recurrence negligible if the infection is cured
Haemorrhage	20% over 5–10 years
Perforation	10% over 5–10 years
Pyloric stenosis	Rare (<1% over 5–10 years)

Table 7. Complications of duodenal ulcers.

conjunction with the widespread use of anticoagulants and anti-platelet therapy for risk reduction of cardiovascular disease.

Gastric ulcers (Figure 6)

Gastric ulcers are less common than duodenal ulcers in those aged less than 40 years but become more common in the elderly. While most gastric ulcers are benign, it is essential to keep in mind that a small percentage may represent an ulcerated gastric cancer. Unlike duodenal ulcers, it is mandatory to biopsy all gastric ulcers or, if not possible at the time of initial endoscopy (e.g. due to active bleeding or a coagulopathy), to ensure that

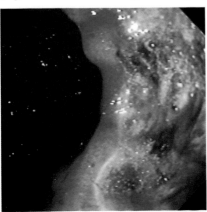

Figure 6. Gastric ulcer. Reproduced with permission from Allison MC. *Self-Assessment Picture Tests: Gastroenterology*. London: Mosby, 1997; p. 8.

Clinical features of gastric versus duodenal ulcers		
	Duodenal	**Gastric**
Age	Young	Elderly
Gender	Male > Female	Equal
Epigastric pain	Hunger or nocturnal	Post-prandial
Vomiting	Uncommon	Common
Anorexia	Uncommon	Common
Weight	Stable	Some weight loss

Table 8. Clinical features of gastric versus duodenal ulcers.

the ulcers have completely healed 8–12 weeks after treatment, at which time the ulcers must be biopsied.

The clinical features of gastric ulcers again fall within the spectrum of peptic ulcer disease in general, although there are some specific symptoms that seem to be more commonly encountered. Table 8 compares and contrasts the clinical features seen in gastric versus duodenal ulcers.

The causes of gastric ulcers are more heterogeneous than duodenal ulcers. Table 9 lists different types of gastric ulcers.

Complications of gastric ulcers

The main complications are similar to those of duodenal ulcers, namely bleeding, perforation and pyloric stenosis (with pyloric channel ulcers). The often-quoted risk of malignant change in the older literature is not correct: gastric cancer diagnosed at the site of a benign ulcer reflects a misdiagnosis of the initial ulcer. Ulcerated early gastric cancer can respond to acid inhibitory therapy, which complicates matters and necessitates endoscopic follow up of all gastric ulcers to ensure full healing.

NSAID-related gastrointestinal disorders

Non-steroidal anti-inflammatory drugs (NSAIDs) represent one of the most widely prescribed class of medications in the world. Over 35 million NSAID prescriptions and billions of over-the-counter preparations are sold annually in the USA, with equivalent figures for the UK. Half of these prescriptions are

Clinical spectrum of gastric ulcers	
Type of ulcer	**Comment**
Lesser curve	Most common, usually benign.
Greater curve	Suspicion of malignancy.
Giant ulcers	>2.5 cm, usually associated with NSAID use and carry no enhanced risk of malignancy.
Antral ulcers	20% are malignant.
Pre-pyloric ulcers	Behave physiologically like duodenal ulcers, i.e. associated with high acid output.
Pyloric channel ulcers	Anorexia, vomiting and weight loss are common features.
Gastroduodenal ulcers	Usually due to NSAIDs but occasionally seen in *H. pylori* infection, or rarely in Zollinger–Ellison syndrome. Bleeding risk is much higher.

Table 9. Clinical spectrum of gastric ulcers.

given to patients over the age of 60 and 15% of elderly people are taking NSAIDs at any one time.[29] Although the overwhelming majority of patients receiving NSAIDs report no major problems, a significant minority present with dyspepsia and some develop serious GI complications. A meta-analysis evaluating alternative dyspepsia definitions was carried out by Straus *et al.* and concluded that NSAIDs increased the risk of dyspepsia by 36%.[30] The Centers for Disease Control reported in 1984 that between 100,000 and 200,000 hospitalizations and 10,000 to 20,000 deaths occurred annually in the USA as a result of NSAID GI toxicity.[31] The equivalent figure for the UK is 1200 deaths per year.[32]

The increasing use of low dose aspirin for cardiovascular protection is becoming an important cause of NSAID-induced GI damage. This is particularly the case when aspirin is combined with anticoagulants such as warfarin. The introduction of highly selective inhibitors of cyclo-oxygenase (COX)-2 has reduced the magnitude of this problem, but ulcers and ulcer complications will continue to occur in patients treated with this new class.

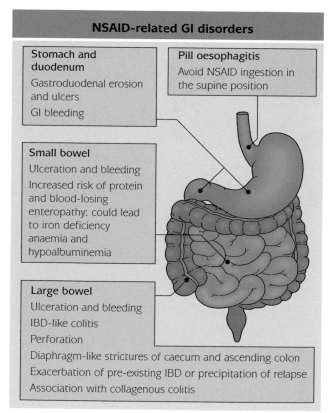

NSAID-related GI disorders

Stomach and duodenum
Gastroduodenal erosion and ulcers
GI bleeding

Pill oesophagitis
Avoid NSAID ingestion in the supine position

Small bowel
Ulceration and bleeding
Increased risk of protein and blood-losing enteropathy; could lead to iron deficiency anaemia and hypoalbuminemia

Large bowel
Ulceration and bleeding
IBD-like colitis
Perforation
Diaphragm-like strictures of caecum and ascending colon
Exacerbation of pre-existing IBD or precipitation of relapse
Association with collagenous colitis

Figure 7. NSAID-related GI disorders. IBD, inflammatory bowel disease.

Spectrum of NSAID gastrointestinal damage

NSAIDs can cause injury throughout the GI tract and liver. Most of these complications can present as vague dyspeptic symptoms and are therefore worthy of note. Figure 7 summarizes the main GI complications of NSAIDs and Figure 8 shows an example of the histological damage caused by NSAIDs (chemical gastritis).

Risk factors for development of NSAID-related gastroduodenal ulcers

Generally speaking, the risk of gastroduodenal mucosal injury is increased in elderly patients with significant co-morbid

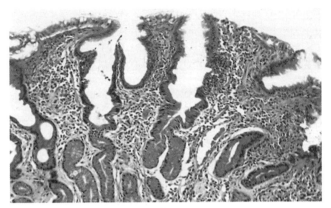

Figure 8. Chemical gastritis, e.g. NSAID-induced, biliary or alcohol. Reproduced with permission from Stevens A, Lowe JS, Young B. *Wheater's Basic Histopathology*, 4th Edition. Edinburgh: Churchill Livingstone, 2002; p. 137.

Risk factors for NSAID ulcers
Age > 60 years
Previous ulcer
Concomitant use of corticosteroids
Concomitant use of anticoagulants
Multiple NSAIDs or NSAID + aspirin
Short-term use of NSAID (<2 weeks)
Serious co-morbid disease or major surgery
Concomitant infection with *H. pylori*
Cigarette smoking
Ethanol abuse

Table 10. Risk factors for NSAID ulcers.

disease who require short-term NSAID therapy (Table 10). Both the dose and the type of NSAID also influence the risk of damage. A meta-analysis by Henry *et al.* showed that, overall, ibuprofen was associated with the lowest relative risk, followed by diclofenac. Azapropazone, tolmetin, ketoprofen and piroxicam ranked highest for risk, and indomethacin, naproxen, sulindac and aspirin occupied intermediate positions.[33]

Complications of NSAID ulcers

The spectrum of complications is similar to that of peptic ulcers not associated with NSAIDs. However, the risk of bleeding and perforation is higher and the risk of pyloric stenosis is lower.

Management of peptic ulcer disease

General measures

- Stop smoking.
- Reduce alcohol intake.
- Eat sensibly: there is no need to institute a special diet but patients clearly have to avoid food items that exacerbate their symptoms. Regular meals can help control of symptoms.
- If NSAIDs are involved, prevention is better than cure. Thus, these drugs should be avoided in patients with two or three of the risk factors for ulcer complications. If they are prescribed in patients with high risk, prophylactic acid inhibition or cytoprotection should be given. If complications develop despite the initial caution and safeguards, the NSAID has to be stopped until complete healing occurs and a long-term management plan is instituted.

H. pylori-positive peptic ulcers

If peptic ulcer patients are found to have *H. pylori* infection, this should be eradicated in all types of ulcers. The specific eradication regimes will be discussed at length later in the book. Though eradication of *H. pylori* infection on its own is enough to heal most peptic ulcers, there are situations when the use of additional healing agents is necessary. These are listed below.

Complicated ulcers: for example ulcers that bleed require additional healing agents, such as acid inhibitory drugs, until the lesions are fully healed. In our unit, we initiate eradication therapy in all patients with *H. pylori*-positive duodenal and gastric ulcers who present to the hospital with GI bleeding. We continue acid inhibitory therapy for a total of 8 weeks, and prefer to use a proton pump inhibitor (PPI) for acid inhibition in these patients. The long-term management of duodenal versus gastric ulcers is outlined in Figure 9.

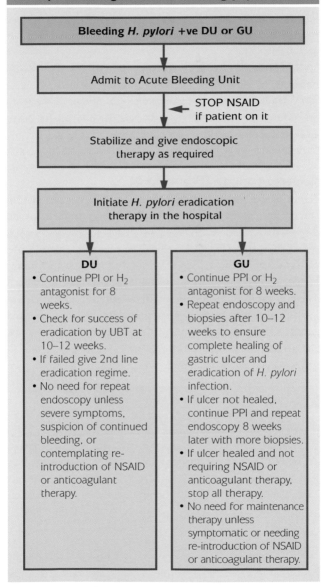

Hospital management of bleeding peptic ulcers

Bleeding *H. pylori* +ve DU or GU

↓

Admit to Acute Bleeding Unit

↓ ← STOP NSAID if patient on it

Stabilize and give endoscopic therapy as required

↓

Initiate *H. pylori* eradication therapy in the hospital

↓

DU
- Continue PPI or H₂ antagonist for 8 weeks.
- Check for success of eradication by UBT at 10–12 weeks.
- If failed give 2nd line eradication regime.
- No need for repeat endoscopy unless severe symptoms, suspicion of continued bleeding, or contemplating re-introduction of NSAID or anticoagulant therapy.

GU
- Continue PPI or H₂ antagonist for 8 weeks.
- Repeat endoscopy and biopsies after 10–12 weeks to ensure complete healing of gastric ulcer and eradication of *H. pylori* infection.
- If ulcer not healed, continue PPI and repeat endoscopy 8 weeks later with more biopsies.
- If ulcer healed and not requiring NSAID or anticoagulant therapy, stop all therapy.
- No need for maintenance therapy unless symptomatic or needing re-introduction of NSAID or anticoagulant therapy.

Figure 9. Hospital management of bleeding peptic ulcers.

In the case of duodenal ulcers, we bring the patients back 10–12 weeks after the initial therapy for a urea breath test (UBT) to ensure that the infection has been successfully eradicated. If not, we institute a second line eradication regime, and repeat the assessment.

NSAID and other *H. pylori*-negative ulcers: these could be healed by H_2 antagonists, PPIs or misoprostil. The balance of evidence in recent years has swung in favour of the more powerful PPIs and H_2 antagonists (see Appendix 1 for doses and duration of treatment; e.g. ranitidine 150 mg twice daily, or cimetidine 400 mg).

Gastric cancer (Figure 10)

Gastric cancer remains a major health problem, being the fourth commonest cause of cancer death in Europe.[34] In the USA, an estimated 21,700 new diagnoses were made in 2001 and 12,800 patients were expected to die in the same year.[35] On a global scale, gastric cancer remains the world's second commonest malignancy, having only been overtaken by lung cancer in the late 1980s.[36] There is substantial international variation in gastric cancer incidence, with the highest rates reported from Korea, Japan and eastern Asia. Other high incidence areas include Eastern Europe and parts of Latin America, while Western Europe and the US generally have low incidence rates.[36] Despite the worldwide

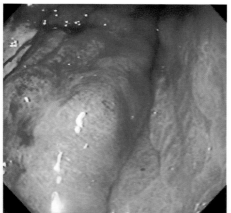

Figure 10. Gastric cancer. Reproduced with permission from Allison MC. *Self-Assessment Picture Tests: Gastroenterology*. London: Mosby, 1997; p. 18.

decline in incidence and the major improvements in diagnosis and treatment, less than 20% of patients are alive at 5 years.

Fear of gastric cancer is one of the main reasons why patients with dyspepsia present to their general practitioner and why most practitioners opt for invasive investigations such as endoscopy. However, in most Western countries including Britain and the USA, the risk of gastric cancer is extremely low in patients under the age of 55 years presenting with new onset dyspepsia. Gastric cancer is found in less than 2% of all cases referred for endoscopy. Early gastric cancer comprises less than 10% of cancer cases in the West, but it is important to diagnose because it is potentially curable (90% 5-year survival) and 60–90% of patients initially present with dyspepsia. Furthermore, "alarm symptoms" such as weight loss, dysphagia, and anaemia help to identify those who need to be investigated in order to exclude malignancy, although between 15% and 50% of dyspeptic patients with gastric cancer do not have these symptoms. Endoscopic evaluation is therefore recommended in older patients presenting with new dyspeptic symptoms and in all patients with alarm symptoms.

The vast majority of gastric cancers are sporadic. However, there is strong evidence that occasional cases have an inherited component with certain families, most notably that of Napoleon Bonaparte, exhibiting a strikingly high incidence of the condition. It is well documented by autopsy that the exiled Emperor had a malignant gastric ulcer complicated by a chronic perforation and haemorrhage. His father, Charles Bonaparte, died from scirrhous carcinoma of the pylorus at the age of 39, and his grandfather, Joseph Bonaparte, also died of "suspected" gastric cancer at the age of 40. At least one of his brothers and one of his sisters also died of the same malignancy. Lending support to the genetic aetiological hypothesis is the recognition that patients with hereditary non-polyposis colon cancer and familial adenomatous polyposis are at an increased risk of developing malignancy in the stomach. Although the genetic gastric cancer link seems strong in some families, the majority of cases are sporadic and have been linked to the chronic inflammation induced by *H. pylori* infection, as will be discussed later.

Pathogenesis

The pathogenesis of gastric cancer represents a classic example of gene–environment interactions. For many decades it was well established that the cancer developed in well-defined histological and pathophysiological stages, with chronic inflammation with gastric atrophy being the most important pathological entity and hypochlorhydria being the most important physiological abnormality. Diets high in food preservatives such as salts and nitrates are thought to contribute to gastric malignancy whereas increased consumption of food containing natural anti-oxidants such as fresh fruit and vegetables may prevent the disease. Alcohol and smoking are thought to contribute to the aetiology. Achlorhydria, pernicious anaemia and blood group A are also associated with a higher risk of gastric malignancy.

The discovery of *Helicobacter pylori* infection in the early 1980s has proved a turning point in understanding the pathogenesis of this malignancy. While the link between *H. pylori* and PUD was established soon after successful culture of the bacterium, the association with gastric cancer lagged almost a decade before credible evidence was presented. The major reason for this delay was inability to demonstrate the presence of active infection in gastric tissue of cancer patients. A major advance in this field came with the recognition that chronic *H. pylori* infection induces physiological and morphological changes within the gastric milieu that increase the risk of neoplastic transformation (Figure 11). It is widely accepted that chronic *H. pylori* infection induces hypochlorhydria and gastric atrophy, both of which are precursors of gastric cancer. These abnormalities, which are well described by the famous Correa hypothesis of gastric carcinogenesis, lead to intestinal metaplasia and dysplasia, and in time to gastric cancer. Presence of the infection in the final stages of this cascade is therefore not necessary for cancer to develop as irreversible damage has already occurred.

Clinical features

The introduction of mass screening programmes in Japan in the 1960s has allowed the detection of very early lesions in which the tumour was limited to the mucosa and submucosa. Eighty percent of patients with early gastric cancer are asymptomatic. Ten percent have peptic ulcer symptoms and there are a number of other non-specific features such as nausea, anorexia or early satiety. A symptomatic presentation is almost by definition indicative of advanced stage, and unfortunately this is the usual mode of presentation in the West. In Western countries, the commonest presenting symptoms are weight loss, abdominal pain, nausea and vomiting, anorexia and dysphagia. Most of these symptoms are non-specific and are very common in elderly patients for other reasons. As a result, late presentation is a particular problem in older patients, and requires a high level of suspicion.

In some studies 40% of patients will have had symptoms for <3 months but 60% will have been symptomatic for 3 months or longer and up to 20% for over 1 year. The late presentation of the disease probably explains why its prognosis remains so dismal, with only 10% of patients being alive at 5 years.

The clinical manifestations also depend critically on the anatomical location of the tumour. Large tumours in the fundus and body may simply manifest with occult blood loss. In contrast, tumours of the antrum can delay gastric emptying and lead to early satiety, anorexia and eventually the features of

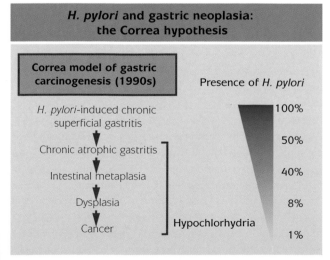

Figure 11. *H. pylori* and gastric neoplasia: the Correa hypothesis.

gastric outlet obstruction. Tumours of the proximal stomach may involve the distal oesophagus and present with dysphagia. What is often more surprising, however, is the considerable size gastric tumours may reach before becoming symptomatic.

As might be anticipated, presentation with local or distant metastatic disease is frequent. Local spread is usually to local and regional nodes but occasionally lymphatic spread will involve more distant nodes such as the supraclavicular (Virchow's) node or the rare umbilical (Sister Mary Joseph's) nodule. More advanced local spread may involve the omentum, pancreas and even the transverse colon. In advanced gastric cancer up to 90% of patients present with local spread and this can make radical resection a formidable undertaking, particularly in elderly malnourished patients. Distant spread to the liver, lungs and bone is very common but peritoneal spread and malignant ascites can also occur.

Diagnosis

Diagnosis of gastric cancer is straightforward, particularly in advanced cases, but may require a high index of suspicion, and a careful history and examination are therefore very essential. Whilst the presence of weight loss, a sucussion splash or a mass in the epigastrium are clearly suggestive of gastric cancer, no single presentation is unique to the disease. More typically the history may be non-specific with loss of appetite, weight loss, abdominal pain and other vague symptoms. Physical examination is frequently unrewarding even in advanced gastric cancer.

Blood tests

A hypochromic, microcytic anaemia is a common finding and the FOB test may be positive, although again this does not localize the source of blood loss and is rarely diagnostic on its own. Liver function test results may be abnormal in advanced disease, and both the C-reactive protein (C-RP) and erythrocyte sedimentation rate (ESR) may be elevated, but all of these findings can occur in other contexts, particularly in elderly patients. For these reasons, some form of examination of the upper GI tract is indicated if gastric carcinoma is suspected.

Endoscopy

Upper GI endoscopy has been shown to be more accurate than barium radiology in the diagnosis of gastric cancer. The principle advantage of endoscopy is its ability to allow close inspection of the mucosa, which is generally the only circumstance under which early gastric carcinoma is found, but more importantly to allow biopsy and a firm histological diagnosis to be made. Gastric carcinoma is usually obvious at endoscopy, either due to gross distortion of the stomach or the presence of an obvious polypoid mass. Certain presentations are more difficult. Firstly, it is well recognized that gastric cancer can present as a typical gastric ulcer. For this reason gastric ulcers should always be biopsied unless there are obvious contra-indications. It is also good practice to follow gastric ulceration to healing, with repeated biopsy if required as acid suppressing drugs such as H_2 blockers or PPIs can produce temporary healing of malignant ulcers. Finally, NSAIDs, which are frequently prescribed in the elderly, can produce large malignant appearing ulcers.

Diffuse gastric carcinoma presenting as a "leather bottle" stomach may also be difficult to diagnose at endoscopy. The gastric mucosa itself may not appear particularly abnormal, but an experienced endoscopist may become aware of a different "feel" to the stomach or of a failure to produce normal insufflation. Mucosal biopsies may not be diagnostic because the carcinoma is infiltrative. Under these circumstances a double contrast barium meal demonstrating abnormal motility, or computed tomography scanning confirming a thickened wall, may be helpful.

Finally, examination of the post-operative stomach may present particular difficulties. As previously indicated, surgery for benign ulcer disease was a common operation until the late 1960s when H_2 blockers became available. The cohort of patients who received surgery has now aged, and with the typical lead-in time for gastric carcinoma being 30 years, malignancy may not appear until the 7th or 8th decade. A variety of procedures were in common use including antrectomy and gastroenterostomy (Polya gastrectomy), antrectomy and primary anastomosis (Billroth I partial gastrectomy), vagotomy and pyloroplasty, and vagotomy and gastroenterostomy. Achieving adequate inflation of the stomach in patients with a gastroenterostomy may be difficult. In addition bile reflux gastritis is common and may produce a fragile and mottled mucosa. The appearance of cancer around the margins of a gastroenterostomy may, therefore, be difficult to determine and requires particular vigilance.

Multiple biopsies are essential for diagnosis. As mentioned previously, gastric atrophy and intestinal metaplasia are common findings in elderly patients. The presence of high grade dysplasia, however, should always be regarded as significant because it may indicate a high risk of malignant transformation, or it may reflect the presence of adjacent malignancy.

Gastro-oesophageal reflux disease (GORD)

Definitions and epidemiology

GORD is defined as any symptomatic condition or histopathological change caused by retrograde flow of gastro-duodenal contents across an incompetent gastro-oesophageal junction into the oesophagus. GORD patients can be divided into three main groups:

- GORD patients with oesophagitis (endoscopically evident lesions in the oesophageal mucosa).
- GORD patients with reflux symptoms and abnormal oesophageal acid exposure during ambulatory 24-hour pH monitoring but with NO endoscopic evidence of oesophagitis (these patients are sometimes labelled as having Endoscopy Negative Reflux Disease or NERD).
- GORD patients with an acid sensitive oesophagus. These form a subset of NERD patients and are characterized by normal oesophageal acid exposure but with a strong correlation between reflux symptoms and gastro-oesophageal reflux events, as revealed during ambulatory 24-hour pH monitoring.

Symptoms of GORD are extremely common and almost all adults in the West will complain of heartburn at some stage.

As mentioned in the introduction, it is possible, and practically desirable, to separate GORD from dyspepsia. The cardinal feature of GORD is frequent heartburn. This is described as a burning sensation in the epigastrium or retrosternal region that characteristically radiates up towards the throat, is precipitated by consuming a large meal, lying flat, stooping, or lifting heavy objects, and is relieved by antacids or acid inhibitory therapy. However, gastro-oesophageal reflux does not always cause symptoms. Although the classic symptoms of heartburn are usually caused by acid reflux, oesophagitis could also be caused by alkaline reflux (refluxate containing bicarbonate, bile and pancreatic enzymes).

GORD affects men and women equally but more men develop oesophagitis than women (ration of 2:1 to 3:1), and for Barrett's metaplasia the ratio is even more impressive (men to women 10:1).[37] Pregnancy seems to be a particular physiological condition that predisposes to GORD, with 48–79% of pregnant women complaining of reflux-like symptoms.[38,39] GORD is also a disease of Caucasians particularly in Europe and North America, with a very small percentage of Asians and Africans developing this condition.[40]

Clinical features of GORD
- Heartburn.
- Regurgitation of acid, bile or food.
- Water brash.
- Dysphagia.
- Excess salivation during pain.
- Chest pain in some patients; could be indistinguishable from angina pectoris.
- Extra-oesophageal symptoms:
  - Cough, wheeze, or sleep apnoea. Nocturnal asthma may be the only feature and this could be cured by appropriate anti-reflux therapy.
  - Globus, sore throat or hoarseness.
  - Bad breath, gingivitis, enamel pits.
  - Early satiety, bloating and nausea.
- GORD may be completely asymptomatic.

Pathogenesis of GORD

The fundamental abnormality in GORD is exposure of oesophageal epithelium to gastric secretions (which may contain duodenal contents as well) that result in either histopathological injury or elicitation of symptoms. Several mechanisms are involved in the pathogenesis of GORD, and these include **motility** and **non-motility** factors.[41] In relation to motility factors, it is well established that GORD is primarily a motor disorder of the upper gastrointestinal tract involving the lower oesophageal sphincter (LOS), oesophageal body, stomach and the antropyloroduodenal anti-reflux mechanism. Several abnormalities of the LOS have been described including decreased resting pressures, abnormal adaptive responses and excessive inappropriate relaxations. Oesophageal abnormalities include uncoordinated contractions and diminished amplitude of peristaltic contractions. Gastric abnormalities that have been described include gastroparesis and gastric dysrhythmia. Finally, excessive bile reflux has been described as a manifestation of abnormal antropyloroduodenal anti-reflux mechanism. Non-motility factors include acid hypersecretion as in patients with gastrinomas (43% of whom have endoscopic abnormalities of the oesophagus)[42] or *H. pylori*-induced duodenal ulcers, bile reflux, decreased salivary or oesophageal bicarbonate secretion, decreased epidermal growth factor and decreased oesophageal mucus.[43]

Role of hiatus hernia

Although the presence of hiatus hernia does not necessarily lead to reflux disease, the presence of the gastro-oesophageal junction in the chest, with its lower intrathoracic pressure, may facilitate reflux and oesophageal damage.

Hiatus hernia is a very common disorder; more than 30% of subjects over the age of 50 have evidence of this abnormality. It is better demonstrated on barium studies but endoscopy allows assessment of oesophagitis and its complications. Hiatus hernias are of three main types: sliding (commonest), rolling (also called para-oesophageal and characterized by dysphagia that is relieved by a change in posture) and incarcerated (classically diagnosed on chest X-ray showing an air–fluid level behind the heart).

Role of dietary factors and medications

Certain food items and beverages are known either to decrease the LOS pressure (e.g. fatty foods, chocolate, alcohol) or to be irritant to the oesophageal mucosa (e.g. citrus fruit, tomatoes and coffee). Among the medications that relax the LOS are anticholinergics, calcium channel blockers and benzodiazepines, while directly irritant drugs include aspirin and other NSAIDs, alendronate sodium, ferrous sulphate and potassium preparations.

Complications of GORD

- Metaplastic change (Barrett's metaplasia) with increased risk of dysplasia and oesophageal adenocarcinoma.
- Stricture formation.
- Ulceration and bleeding.

Investigations of GORD

For obvious reasons, it is not practical or necessary to investigate every patient who presents to their GP with heartburn. A well taken history is usually sufficient to confirm the diagnosis of GORD and to initiate appropriate therapy. The presence of chronic, severe, atypical or alarm symptoms usually drive the patient and GP to seek diagnostic investigations. It is highly unusual, however, for this to happen before a short course of empirical therapy is tried.

Upper GI endoscopy (Figure 12)

This is the best initial diagnostic test. It allows detection and grading of oesophagitis and also detection of any complications such as Barrett's metaplasia, malignancy or stricture formation. While oesophagitis can be detected at endoscopy, over half of patients with true GORD will not have evidence of mucosal damage (NERD). Thus endoscopy is reliable in diagnosing GORD in those who have oesophagitis, but a negative test does not exclude the diagnosis. Oesophageal erythema or the presence of a hiatus hernia are of doubtful significance in terms of diagnosis of GORD. There have been several endoscopic classification schemes for grading of oesophagitis and this has

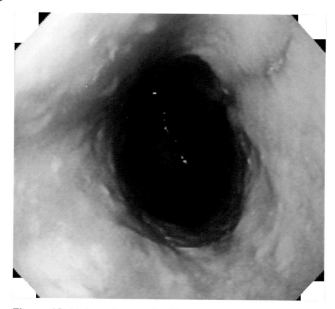

Figure 12. High grade oesophagitis. Reproduced with permission from Allison MC. *Self-Assessment Picture Tests: Gastroenterology*. London: Mosby, 1997; p. 8.

created considerable confusion regarding published trials. In an attempt to harmonize reporting of the severity of oesophagitis, a panel of experts convened a special meeting in 1994 at the World Congress of Gastroenterology which took place in Los Angeles, USA. The panel came up with the so-called Los Angeles endoscopic classification of oesophagitis, which categorizes mucosal injury into four grades (A, B, C and D).[44] This classification perhaps remains the most thoroughly evaluated scheme for oesophagitis and more endoscopists are using it than any other system.

The Los Angeles endoscopic classification system for oesophagitis

- Grade A
  One (or more) mucosal break no longer than 5 mm, that does not extend between the tops of two mucosal folds.

- Grade B
  One (or more) mucosal break more than 5 mm long that does not extend between the tops of two mucosal folds.
- Grade C
  One (or more) mucosal break that is continuous between the tops of two or more mucosal folds but which involves less than 75% of the circumference.
- Grade D
  One (or more) mucosal break which involves at least 75% of the oesophageal circumference

Double contrast barium studies

This is only useful in detecting strictures, oesophageal ulcers or hiatus hernia. It will not diagnose oesophagitis or Barrett's metaplasia, and most gastroenterologists would not use it as a first-line diagnostic test.

Ambulatory 24-hour pH monitoring

This is widely used to establish the presence of excessive gastro-oesophageal reflux and to correlate symptoms temporally with reflux. Despite its limitations, it is still the best available test for quantifying oesophageal acid exposure. The main indication for this test is to document excessive acid reflux in patients without endoscopic evidence of oesophagitis. It is also used to evaluate the efficacy of medical therapy and the need for and response to surgical intervention. For example, very few surgeons would undertake anti-reflux surgery without documented evidence of reflux.

The test is performed by intranasally introducing a thin pH probe and positioning it 5 cm above the proximal margin of the LOS, as determined manometrically. The recording from the probe is stored in digital format in a box fitted to the patient's waist. The patient is then sent home and is asked to conduct his or her daily activities as usual, while recording symptoms, meals (including small snacks and drinks) and any periods of sleep. The percentage of the recording time that the pH is below 4 is known as the **oesophageal acid exposure** and is usually less than 3.5%.[45] However, there is no absolute threshold value that identifies patients with GORD. Twenty five percent of patients with oesophagitis and 30% of those with non-erosive reflux disease have normal oesophageal acid exposure values (see Figure 13A–D).[46]

Oesophageal manometry

Manometry is the standard for diagnosis of motor disorders of the oesophageal body and lower oesophageal sphincter. It has very little to offer in the investigation of dyspepsia or GORD except in excluding such major motor disorders of the oesophagus or in evaluating peristaltic function prior to anti-reflux surgery.

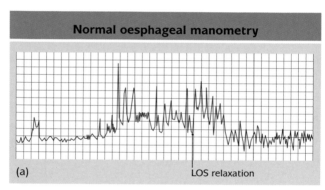

Figure 13. Oesophageal manometry and pH monitoring. (A) Normal oesophageal manometry. This tracing, taken at the level of the lower oesophageal sphincter (LOS), shows a normal resting tone, regular contractions and a relaxation response following deglutition.

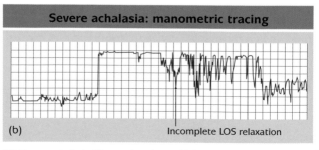

(B) Severe achalasia. The tracing shows high pressure at the LOS, disordered motor contractions and a failure to relax after swallowing.

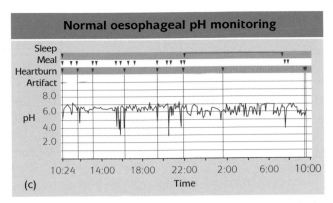

(C) Normal oesophageal pH monitoring. A pH monitoring probe is positioned 5 cm above the LOS. The marks on the top of the graph record periods of symptoms, sleep and meal times over the 24-hour period. Significant acid reflux is defined by a drop in pH below 4. This normal trace demonstrates that a few episodes of mild reflux do occur, but these do not coincide with the patient's symptoms of heartburn.

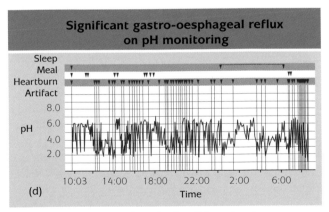

(D) Significant gastro-oesophageal reflux. This tracing demonstrates severe episodes of acid reflux, many of which are prolonged (> 5 minutes); the oesophageal pH is below 4 for about 25% of the total recording time. The reflux is at its worst in the postprandial periods and there is good correlation with the symptoms of heartburn. Reproduced with permission from Aspinall R, Taylor-Robinson S. *Mosby's Color Atlas and Text of Gastroenterology and Liver Disease*. London: Mosby, 2001; pp. 15–16.

Management of GORD

The objectives in treating GORD are based on the following principles:

(1) Reduction in the volume and potency of the gastro-oesophageal refluxate.

(2) Protection of the oesophageal mucosa from acid-induced injury.

(3) Enhancement of oesophageal clearance.

(4) Improvement of the gastro-oesophageal junction anti-reflux mechanisms.

In treating GORD, most practitioners use either a "step-up" or "step-down" strategy, and this initially depends on the severity of the condition. In the step-up regimen, which usually starts in primary care and deals with initial uninvestigated presentations, the patient is given advice about lifestyle modification (see Figures 24 and 25) and given simple antacids or over-the-counter (OTC) medications including H_2 antagonists. If this does not help, the patient is prescribed an H_2 antagonist (healing dose) or a pro-kinetic drug (such as metoclopramide, domperidone or cisapride) and this is usually given for 4 weeks to assess response. Unfortunately, of the patients who are prescribed H_2 antagonists, 40% will not experience relief of their symptoms and up to 60% of those with oesophagitis will not experience full mucosal healing. To achieve higher rates of healing and symptomatic relief, many patients require ever increasing doses of H_2 antagonists, and they will eventually require proton pump inhibitors (PPIs), prescription of which heralds anxiety on the part of the GP. It is usually at that stage that referral to specialists is initiated. Some GPs are reluctant to start patients on powerful acid inhibitory therapy without a diagnosis being made. This concern is entirely justified, as once patients are started on such "wonderful" drugs, they are reluctant to tolerate any symptoms of reflux after the "trial" period is over. It becomes very hard to step down to less effective medication and these patients become long-term users of PPI therapy without ever having an assessment of their upper GI tract. For this reason, many GPs request proper investigation and documentation of GORD before prescribing PPIs.

Once investigations are initiated, a diagnosis of mild to moderate reflux oesophagitis is most commonly treated with a good healing dose of a PPI, given for 4 weeks and followed by half the dose for another 4 weeks. In severe oesophagitis, 8 weeks of high dose PPI is usually needed to ensure full healing. Response is then assessed to decide on so-called maintenance therapy. Maintenance therapy is needed because of the strikingly high relapse rate for GORD following cessation of therapy. In one study in which patients were given omeprazole for 8–12 weeks and then followed up, 60% relapsed at 4 months and 82% at 6 months after omeprazole was stopped.[47,48] This suggests that in patients with documented oesophagitis some form of maintenance therapy is essential, and this decision has to be arrived at carefully with a number of factors taken into consideration. Most important among these are the long-term effects of profound acid inhibition on the gastric mucosa in the presence of *H. pylori* infection as will be discussed later.

The step-up regimen works very well in the context of primary care but there are situations in which this approach is less desirable. If the symptoms are severe, the patient is older than 55, or alarm symptoms are present (e.g. anorexia, weight loss, dysphagia, odynophagia, anaemia, occult blood in the stool, jaundice, or pulmonary symptoms) then the patient should be referred for endoscopy without delay. If symptoms are severe initially or they have been present for a considerable time and had not responded to self-medication with OTC drugs, most practitioners would use high-dose PPIs to assess response. This is the so-called step down regimen, where the most effective medication (PPI) is given first and if the patient responds well, the doctor tries to reduce the strength of this medication, stepping down in the process to a lower dose, given less frequently (e.g. as required dosing) or using an H_2 antagonist or antacid instead.

When to step down treatment
- Mild reflux oesophagitis with recurrent symptoms. These patients could successfully be managed on H_2 antagonists or antacid–alginate mixtures.
- Patients with reflux oesophagitis who were treated with high dose PPI without trying other therapies.

When not to step down

- Erosive, ulcerating or stricturing disease confirmed endoscopically. These patients almost always relapse and it would be more appropriate to maintain them on PPI therapy.
- Patients taking NSAID therapy.
- Severe GORD not maintained by other therapy.
- If previous attempts to step down failed.

The bottom line is that there are no data to show which strategy (step-up or step-down) is better, and indeed step-up could transform into step-down in time. Common sense is often the best strategy.

Concern about long-term PPI therapy

PPIs are very effective drugs that have transformed the management of acid-related disorders. They have an excellent safety record and there have been no major side effects reported since their introduction in the early 1990s. However, concern was raised regarding their effect on the gastric mucosa in the presence of *H. pylori* infection. *H. pylori* induces inflammation of the gastric mucosa that seems to affect the antral part of the stomach more than the acid-producing corpus region, at least in subjects with normal acid secretion. In those in whom acid secretion is reduced, either naturally or pharmacologically (by PPI therapy), the distribution of gastritis changes to that of a severe corpus-predominant pattern and there is evidence that this gastritis progresses to gastric atrophy.[49–51] The concern here is clearly related to the role of gastric atrophy as a precursor lesion for gastric adenocarcinoma. There is no evidence that PPI-induced gastric atrophy will necessarily transform to gastric cancer with the passage of time, but clearly it is advisable to at least reduce this risk by preventing the change in the pattern of gastritis. This could be achieved by eradicating *H. pylori* infection in subjects in whom prolonged PPI therapy is planned or anticipated. PPI therapy exerts no effect on gastric mucosa of *H. pylori*-negative subjects. The concerns about long-term PPI therapy discussed here form the basis for the recommendation that all such patients should be tested for *H. pylori* infection and given eradication if found to be positive.

Surgery for GORD

If all medical therapy fails, the final option might be to consider a surgical solution. Clearly the patient evaluation would include documented evidence of GORD, including 24-hour pH monitoring. The patient must present a good operative risk and the surgical procedure has to be explained thoroughly to the patient, including an explanation of the potential side effects, which could be considerable (dysphagia, gas bloating, flatulence and diarrhoea). The mortality rate was reported at 0.2% among 2453 patients.[52] In expert hands and in centres where these procedures are carried out routinely, the outcome is usually very favourable. The advent of laparoscopic surgery has narrowed the choice of procedure to two main operations: laparoscopic Nissen (360-degree) fundoplication and the Toupet (270-degree) fundoplication. Fundoplication attempts to correct the underlying mechanical and physiological abnormalities of GORD.

Who is fundoplication FOR?

- Failed medical therapy with troublesome symptomatic oesophagitis.
- Successful medical therapy in a young patient unwilling to take or intolerant of long-term PPI therapy (see above).
- Persistent symptoms due to regurgitation (asthma, bronchiectasis, laryngitis).

Who is NOT a candidate for fundoplication?

- Elderly patients with co-morbid disease and poor surgical risk.
- Symptomatic patients without quantifiable abnormal reflux.
- Patients with concomitant functional dyspepsia (bloating, early satiety, etc.) whose symptoms could be made worse by fundoplication.
- Patients with poor oesophageal peristaltic function who are at risk of developing severe dysphagia with fundoplication.

Cholelithiasis

Ultrasonography of a normal population will detect gallstones in 10–15%, and these become more common with advancing age. The majority of gallstones remain asymptomatic, but 15% of patients present with "biliary" symptoms, particularly when complications occur. Biliary colic, which is caused by impaction of a gallstone, is characterized by severe, episodic and constant (rather than colicky) pain in the epigastrium or right upper quadrant and can last 1 to several hours. This can usually be easily distinguished from the pain or discomfort of functional dyspepsia.

While many patients with gallstones also complain of bloating, nausea and other vague upper abdominal symptoms, these complaints are just as common in patients without gallstones. Moreover, cholecystectomy does not reliably result in long-term relief of any of these vague complaints and therefore is not recommended. Cholecystectomy in a patient with non-biliary type pain is likely to result in the patient at a later date being labelled as having the post-cholecystectomy syndrome.

Functional Dyspepsia

In approximately 50% of investigated dyspeptic patients, either no abnormalities or minor abnormalities (such as gastric erythema or a few gastric erosions) are found at endoscopy. These patients are labelled as having functional dyspepsia (FD), a diagnosis of exclusion.[53]

Pathogenesis of functional dyspepsia

The pathogenesis of FD remains uncertain. Half the patients have *H. pylori*-induced gastritis, but this is also common in asymptomatic subjects. There are no symptoms that are specific to *H. pylori*-infected patients. Gastric acid secretion is known to be increased in a small subgroup of patients with FD,[54] but acid levels are normal in the majority.

In FD patients, gastric and duodenal sensations are disturbed.[53] In about half of patients distension induces symptoms at lower pressures or volumes than it does in healthy people,[53] and in a quarter to a half of FD patients there is delayed gastric emptying. In addition, a subset of patients have altered intragastric distribution of food, which reflects abnormal proximal gastric relaxation (a "stiff" fundus).[53] Some FD patients have features suggestive of irritable bowel syndrome (IBS). About a third have an erratic disturbance of defecation closely linked to abdominal pain, and may therefore have genuine IBS. There is evidence that the gut is hypersensitive in both FD and IBS patients.[53]

While smoking and alcohol seem less important in FD, there is evidence that coffee consumption exacerbates symptoms. As would be expected, psychosocial factors have an important role in FD. FD patients are more likely to present with anxiety and affective disorders such as depression compared with patients without FD.

Investigations of functional dyspepsia

These come under the same category of investigating dyspepsia generally. There is a limit to how far investigations should be taken before accepting a diagnosis of FD. The aim is to achieve confidence about exclusion of the commonest organic causes of dyspepsia.

Investigation versus testing for *H. pylori*

A careful and detailed clinical history with an informed approach to testing is necessary. There is wide agreement that patients older than 55 years or those with alarm features warrant prompt referral for endoscopy and further investigations as indicated. *H. pylori* testing will aid subsequent management in the remainder of patients.

There are two main strategies to deal with patients who are found to have *H. pylori* infection. The first is the "Test and scope" strategy, which allows one to find out which patients have PUD and which have FD, the two most frequent diagnoses in this context. In addition, it also allows the diagnosis of oesophageal conditions such as oesophagitis and Barrett's metaplasia. However, these conditions are best treated with therapy directed at symptom control, because treatment directed at healing does not prevent complications or decrease the recognised additional risk of oesophageal adenocarcinoma. The second strategy is "Test and treat", where eradication therapy is given without finding out what the actual diagnosis is. This strategy involves testing for *H. pylori* by breath test or serology, followed by *H. pylori* eradication in cases with *H. pylori* and symptomatic therapy for the remainder. A number of management trials have been published that demonstrate that the strategy is as effective as endoscopy in determining therapy for dyspepsia. Such a strategy will cover the following situations:

- Provide appropriate treatment for PUD, including reduction of relapse, bleeding, perforation and gastric outlet obstruction.

- Provide cure for a small but significant group of patients with *H. pylori*-associated FD (see later).
- Reduce concerns about worsening gastritis and developing gastric atrophy during treatment of GORD with PPIs and potentially could reduce gastric cancer risk.

On the other hand, a "Test and treat" strategy will expose more patients to broad spectrum antibiotics, but there are no other known significant disadvantages of such an approach. Recent trials suggest that "test and treat" is a safe and cost effective strategy that produces similar long-term outcomes to a strategy based on endoscopy. The effectiveness of this strategy will need to be re-assessed if the prevalence of *H. pylori* falls to very much lower levels than at present (for example in parts of North America). However, we are convinced by the substantial evidence base that this approach is both cost effective and safe, and most clinicians now favour a "*H. pylori* test and treat" strategy for uncomplicated dyspepsia in patients under 55.

Principles of management

As with the management of any medical condition, it is important to keep the patients fully informed about their illness, its pathogenesis, potential outcome and realistic expectations. In this manner, the patient feels part of the decision making process and appreciates the limitations of medical knowledge. Reassurance is extremely important in the context of FD. A considerable number of patients have anxiety about serious illness and cancer in particular. It is very important to reassure the patients that they do not have cancer or a condition that can lead to malignancy. Dietary advice is also important, particularly in patients in whom symptoms are induced by certain food items or beverages: for example, high consumption of tea or coffee, and high fat diets that exacerbate reflux and cause delayed gastric emptying. Advice about stopping certain medications that cause dyspepsia may also be appropriate.

Initial treatment

Most practitioners start with a short (4 week) therapeutic trial with an acid inhibitor. H_2 antagonists are widely used as first-line drugs, but their modest effects in FD have led to their substitution by PPIs that are more efficacious in the context of FD. If the patient complains of a predominant symptom, this may aid the physician in selecting the initial medication and in predicting the possible response to treatment.

If the patient fails to respond to acid inhibitory therapy after 4 weeks, it is reasonable either to increase the dose or to switch

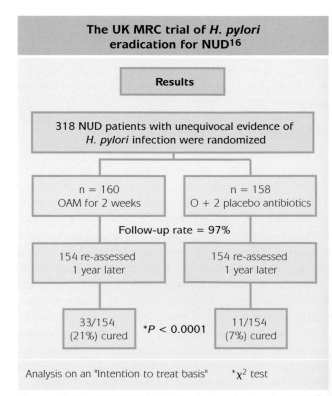

Figure 14. The UK MRC Trial of *H. pylori* eradication for NUD.[16] OAM, omeprazole + amoxicillin + metronidazole; O, omeprazole.

to an alternative or even consider a prokinetic drug. Failure to respond after 8 weeks usually prompts referral for specialist evaluation.

Eradicating *H. pylori* infection cures FD in a small subgroup of patients. The best results were demonstrated by the UK MRC Trial of *H. pylori* eradication for NUD (Figure 14). This trial was based in the West of Scotland, an area with a high prevalence of *H. pylori* and PUD. Results have been replicated in other areas of the world with a similar background prevalence of both conditions (e.g. Ireland), but the results have been less impressive in countries with a low background prevalence of *H. pylori* and PUD. A meta-analysis has suggested a small therapeutic gain over 12 months of follow up (15 cases needed to be treated to cure one case).

Initial management of functional dyspepsia

- Try to make an informed clinical diagnosis.
- Avoid unnecessary investigations and go for the test that is most likely to be informative.
- Consider psychosocial factors at this early stage and try to understand the patient's perspectives.
- Always keep the patient fully informed and reassured.

Long term management

By its nature, FD is a relapsing and remitting condition. The clinician must avoid prolonged treatment and must encourage the patient to try to "come off" the prescribed medications, at least for a period of time. In patients with resistant symptoms, it is reasonable to try antispasmodic or antidepressant therapy. However, this form of therapy usually comes after traditional therapy has failed and after specialist referral has already taken place. We find that referral to a clinical psychologist/psychiatrist with a special interest in functional bowel disorders is an excellent adjunct to our own management of these patients. Quite frequently, these resistant cases are helped significantly by some form of behavioural therapy or psychotherapy.

Treatment for functional dyspepsia[53]

Initial treatment

- Acid inhibitory therapy (H_2 receptor antagonist, PPI) or
- Prokinetic drug (domperidone) if the above treatment fails
- Switch treatment if first drug type fails

Resistant cases (failed initial treatment)

- *H. pylori* eradication
- Sucralfate or bismuth (doubtful benefit but may work in patients with biliary or other types of non-*H. pylori* gastritis)
- Antispasmodics (e.g. mebeverine)
- Antidepressants (e.g. selective serotonin reuptake inhibitor or tricyclic drug)
- Behavioural therapy or psychotherapy

Helicobacter pylori *Infection*

The *Helicobacter* genus consists of at least 24 species found in the GI tracts of animals and humans.[55] One of these species is *Helicobacter pylori* (*H. pylori*), a gram negative, spiral shaped, microaerophilic, urease-positive bacillus (Figure 15), which is known to chronically infect the stomachs of over half the world's population. The infection is acquired during childhood, most probably via the faecal/oral or gastric/oral routes, and if not treated with antibiotics, will persist throughout life.[56] The organism is 2.5–5 micrometers long with 4–6 unipolar flagellae. These flagellae are thought to allow it to move through the mucus layer within the stomach and come to reside between this layer and the gastric epithelium. Eighty percent of the bacilli are free living; however, the remainder are attached to epithelial cells. Once attached the organism induces ultra-structural changes in gastric epithelial cells. Although the bacteria mainly reside on the surface mucus gel layer with little invasion of the gastric glands, the host responds with an impressive humoral and cell-mediated immune response (Figure 16). This immune response is largely ineffective, however, as most infections become chronically established with little evidence that spontaneous clearance occurs.

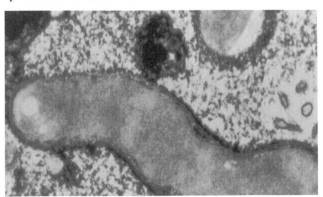

Figure 15. Electron microscope picture of *H. pylori*.

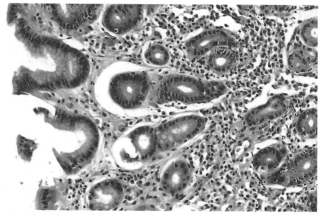

Figure 16. *H. pylori*-induced gastritis. Reproduced with permission from Stevens A, Lowe JS, Young B. *Wheater's Basic Histopathology*, 4th Edition. Edinburgh: Churchill Livingstone, 2002; p. 137.

In order to overcome the inhospitable and acidic gastric environment, *H. pylori* is equipped with several factors that allow it to colonize and evade the host defences, including the immune response. *H. pylori* possesses a urease enzyme that allows it to hydrolyse gastric urea into ammonia and carbon dioxide. This permits *H. pylori* to maintain a constant internal and periplasmic pH, even in the presence of a very high external H^+ concentration. In addition, *H. pylori* expresses a urea transport protein (UreI) with unique acid-dependent properties that activates the rate of urea entry into the cytoplasm. The combination of a neutral pH-optimum urease and an acid-regulated urea channel explains why *H. pylori* is unique in its ability to inhabit the human stomach.[57,58] Indeed, isogenic urease-negative mutants of *H. pylori* are incapable of colonizing the gastric mucosa.[59] While *H. pylori* is well equipped to colonize such an inhospitable environment, it is essentially a neutralophile, that grows best at a pH of between 6.0 and 8.0. In order to conserve energy and resources, *H. pylori* seeks out a niche that does not constantly challenge its acid-resisting and acid-adaptation machinery. This explains why the initial colonization is maximal in the antral part of the stomach, a region with a higher pH than the acid-producing corpus mucosa. This also explains why the distribution of the infection changes when gastric acid secretion is inhibited by pharmacological means. In these circumstances, *H. pylori* and its associated inflammation spread to involve the hitherto protected corpus mucosa. This has a very important consequence in relation to gastric cancer risk, as will be discussed later.

H. pylori possesses a variety of other virulence factors. The best characterized is the *cag* pathogenicity island (cag-PAI), a 40 kb chromosomal DNA, which contains approximately 31 genes.[60,61] Several of the genes present on the cag-PAI encode components of a type IV secretion system, which allows CagA (cytotoxin-associated gene A), a 120–130kDa protein product, and other bacterial proteins encoded by the cag-PAI to be injected into the epithelial cell cytosol. After entering the cell, CagA is phosphorylated and binds to tyrosine phosphatase, which induces secretion of interleukin (IL)-8, a potent chemotactic and activating factor for neutrophils, by the activation of nuclear factor (NF)-κB complexes.[62,63] The cag-PAI also induces cell-surface remodelling, including the induction of pedestal formation, activation of the transcription factor activator protein (AP)-1 and expression of the proto-oncogenes c-*fos* and c-*jun* by activation of the extracellular signal-regulated kinase (ERK)/mitogen-activated protein (MAP) kinase cascade. *H. pylori* strains that do not contain the cag-PAI or possess mutated *cag* genes do not induce these changes or do so to a much lesser extent.

H. pylori strains can be divided into two groups based on the presence/absence of the cag-PAI: type 1 strains, which possess the cag-PAI, and type 2, which do not. Type 1 strains are associated with severe gastritis, peptic ulcer disease, gastric atrophy and non-cardia gastric cancer, thus linking the presence of PAI to increased virulence.[64–67] It should be noted, however, that not all type 1 isolates contain the entire PAI. Infection with a *cagA*-expressing strain is also associated with reduced apoptosis, whereas infection with a *cagA*-negative strain is associated with increased apoptosis. Therefore *cagA* may act to inhibit gastric epithelial-programmed cell death.

Another *H. pylori* virulence factor is possession of the *vacA* gene, which encodes the expression of a vacuolating cytotoxin, VacA. This has been shown to induce vacuole formation in eukaryotic cells and to stimulate epithelial-cell apoptosis.[66–68] The toxin inserts itself into the epithelial-cell membrane, forming a voltage-dependent channel through which bicarbonate and organic anions can be released. Unlike the cag-PAI, all *H. pylori* strains possess the *vacA* gene, although only approximately 50% of strains express the VacA protein. Differences in expression are due to gene sequence variation.[69] Animal studies have shown that infusion of the VacA protein into the stomach results in gastritis and ulceration. Furthermore, humans infected with VacA-expressing *H. pylori* demonstrate a greater degree of gastritis than non-expressing strains. *H. pylori* infection is invariably associated with elevated gastric epithelial cell proliferation, thought to be a consequence of the epithelial damage.

Diagnostic tests for *H. pylori* infection

H. pylori infection can be diagnosed by demonstrating antibodies to the organism in serum, by showing urease activity in the stomach using breath tests or rapid slide urease tests, or by examination of biopsies by histological staining or culture. Antigen derived from the organism can also be identified in stool samples (for good reviews on the subject consult references 70–76).

Serology

Serological methods rely on the detection of specific anti-*H. pylori* IgG antibody in patient's serum. They are simple, non-invasive and widely available but are not useful in demonstrating successful eradication as detectable antibodies remain in the circulation for up to 2 years after successful eradication of the infection. Some kits provide a rapid result while the patient waits in a clinic or physician's office (the so-called near patient test). Laboratory based tests have a high sensitivity and are useful but they are less accurate (and therefore less specific) than other methods. A meta-analysis of 21 studies with commercially available enzyme-linked immunoabsorbent assay (ELISA) serology kits reported overall sensitivity and specificity rates of 85% and 79%, respectively.[77]

In addition, the Medical Devices Agency of Great Britain tested 588 samples of sera with 16 different commercially available ELISA tests and reported an overall accuracy of the assays of 78% (range 68–82%) for all sera.[78] It is difficult therefore to make an argument for the use of these kits on clinical or economic grounds.

In addition to *H. pylori* IgG serology kits, newer serological kits have been developed to detect antibodies to *H. pylori* virulence proteins CagA or VacA (ELISA, Recombinant ImmunoBlot Assay-RIBA-Western Blot). The use of these is currently restricted to the research setting as an adjunct to characterizing the *H. pylori* status of an individual. It is known that these antibodies persist for longer periods than traditional *H. pylori* IgG antibodies, following either therapeutic eradication of the organism or natural disappearance of the infection in the context of gastric atrophy and intestinal metaplasia.

Urease-dependent diagnostic tests

One of the most important enzymes produced by *H. pylori* is *urease,* which catalyzes the hydrolysis of urea into carbon dioxide and ammonia (Figure 17). Both these by-products have

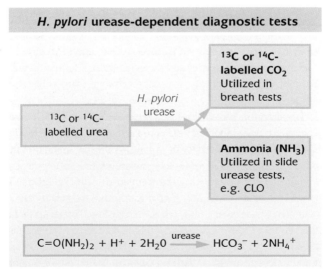

Figure 17. *H. pylori* urease-dependent diagnostic tests.

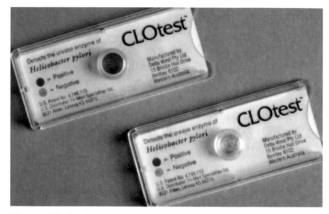

Figure 18. Rapid urease slide test. Purple = positive test; yellow = negative test.

been exploited in designing very accurate diagnostic tests for the organism. The first is the *rapid urease test (RUT)*, an invasive test that relies on the ammonia by-product and requires a gastric mucosal biopsy. The mucosal biopsy is obtained during routine endoscopy and is immediately placed on a slide (CLOtest, Hpfast) or paper (PyloriTek®) impregnated with urea and a pH sensitive indicator (phenol red). If the biopsy harbours *H. pylori* organisms, their urease enzyme will split the urea in the gel or paper and the generation of ammonia will increase the pH, leading to a colour change from yellow to purple (Figure 18).

The reported sensitivities and specificities for RUTs range from 80 to 95% and 95 to 100%, respectively.[79] The sensitivity is dependent on the number of organisms present in the biopsy and it has been reported that 104 organisms are needed to produce a positive test.[80] Increasing the number of mucosal biopsies speeds up the reaction but does not improve the sensitivity.[81] PyloriTek® is read at 1 hour while CLOtest could take up to 24 hours to give a definitive result, suggesting that the former has an advantage in terms of speed.[82] However, experienced practitioners could also read the CLOtest within the first hour and late positives tend to suggest an unusual intragastric environment such as achlorhydria or severe atrophy. The sensitivity and specificity of the RUTs are reduced in patients with upper GI bleeding.[83] It is not clear if this is due to the presence of blood *per se* within the stomach or to some other factor such as concurrent administration of proton pump inhibitors in such patients. Achlorhydria, caused by powerful acid inhibitors or due to severe gastritis and atrophy, is known to give false RUTs.[81] Powerful acid inhibition is associated with a lower *H. pylori* density in the antral region while that in the corpus may be unaffected. For this reason we routinely take biopsies from both antrum and corpus and place them on the same slide to maximize the chances of obtaining a positive result.

The second by-product of the hydrolysis of urea is carbon dioxide and this is utilized in the ***urea breath tests (UBT)***. Urea is labelled with either ^{14}C, which is radioactive, or with the non-radioactive isotope ^{13}C, which is stable and more expensive. In the UBT, the labelled urea is ingested, and in the presence of gastric *H. pylori*, tagged carbon dioxide will be generated in the gastric mucosa and diffuses back to the blood and on to the lungs to be exhaled. A breath sample is taken at baseline before the isotope is ingested and another sample after 20 minutes. Carbon tagged breath tests are of intermediate cost, but are non-invasive. ^{13}C UBTs are available as kits on prescription. These tests can confirm successful eradication but they must be performed when patients are not taking PPIs, bismuth or within 4 weeks of antibiotic use. **The most accurate test for *H. pylori* is the UBT.**

Endoscopic tests

Methods of identifying *H. pylori* that involve endoscopy and biopsy are expensive. Simple biopsy urease tests are a very small additional cost to that of endoscopy. Histology, or culture of the organism add significantly to costs. **Routine use of endoscopy for diagnosis of *H. pylori* is not recommended.**

Faecal antigen tests

These have become available recently but their exact role remains to be determined.

Pathogenesis of *H. pylori* infection

Two-way interaction between *H. pylori* infection and gastric acid secretion

There is accumulating evidence that acid secretory capacity is crucial in determining the distribution and natural history of *H. pylori* infection.[84] *H. pylori* infection is first established in parts of the stomach that have a higher pH such as the antrum (Figures 19 and 20). High acid production by the parietal cells probably protects the corpus mucosa from initial colonization. The antral gastritis is associated with up-regulation of gastrin, the acid stimulatory hormone, and down-regulation of somatostatin, a universal inhibitory GI hormone, with a net effect of increasing the drive for acid secretion. The resultant changes in the acid response are very much dependent on the state and health of

H. pylori infection and gastritis

H. pylori can only colonize gastric type mucosa	It resides in the surface mucous layer and does not penetrate the epithelial layer

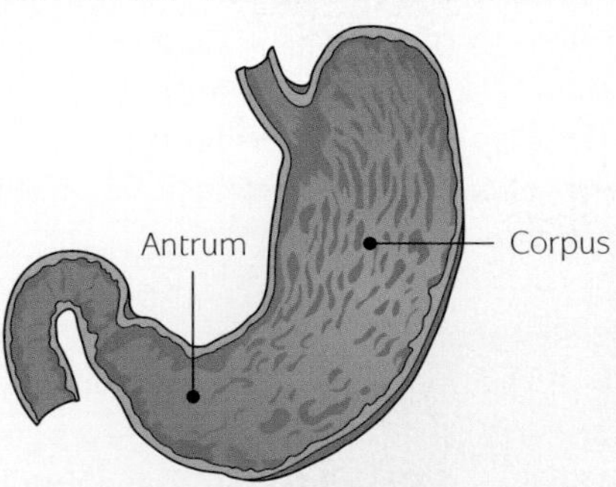

It induces a powerful inflammatory reaction which becomes chronic (**Chronic Gastritis**)

Figure 19. *H. pylori* infection and gastritis.

the corpus mucosa and parietal cell mass. In hosts with low secretory capacity the organism is capable of colonizing a wider niche than would be possible in the presence of high volumes of acid. Colonization of a wider niche including the corpus mucosa leads to further inhibition of acid secretion and a more aggressive gastritis that accelerates the development of gastric atrophy. Once atrophy develops, acid secretion is attenuated not only by the functional inhibition caused by inflammatory mediators such as IL-1β and TNF-α, but also by a more permanent morphological change that is harder to reverse. This situation is very relevant to the subgroup of humans who develop

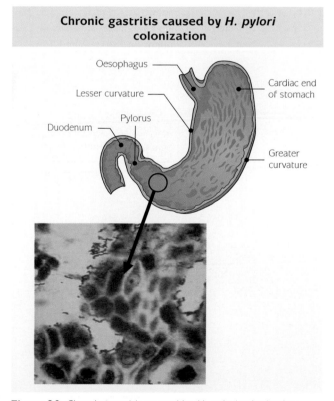

Figure 20. Chronic gastritis caused by *H. pylori* colonization (antrum).

the gastric cancer phenotype in the presence of chronic *H. pylori* infection. The effect of acid secretion on changing the distribution of *H. pylori* colonization and gastritis is most markedly exposed in subjects in whom acid secretion is manipulated by pharmacological means. Thus *H. pylori* infected subjects on long-term PPIs undergo a shift in the pattern of gastritis from antral- to corpus-predominant, and they have a higher risk of developing gastric atrophy, a precursor lesion for gastric neoplasia.[85] This observation provided a clue as to the role of potential endogenous substances that could also inhibit acid secretion, such as IL-1β and TNF-α.

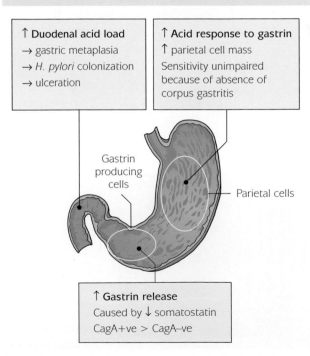

Pathophysiologic abnormalities in duodenal ulcer disease

↑ Duodenal acid load
→ gastric metaplasia
→ *H. pylori* colonization
→ ulceration

↑ Acid response to gastrin
↑ parietal cell mass
Sensitivity unimpaired because of absence of corpus gastritis

Gastrin producing cells

Parietal cells

↑ Gastrin release
Caused by ↓ somatostatin
CagA+ve > CagA−ve

Figure 21. Pathophysiologic abnormalities in duodenal ulcer disease.

In contrast to subjects who are at risk of gastric cancer, subjects who develop duodenal ulcer disease are known to have a large parietal cell mass that is relatively free of *H. pylori*-induced inflammatory activity (Figure 21). This pattern of antral-predominant gastritis with high acid output characterizes the duodenal ulcer diathesis. The high acid output is associated with the development of duodenal gastric metaplasia (DGM), a protective mechanism against the persistent delivery of an increased acid load to the duodenum. The presence of gastric epithelium (DGM) in the duodenum is an invitation for antral *H. pylori* infection to colonize this new niche. The ensuing gastritis, with the production of pro-inflammatory cytokines such as IL-1β and TNF-α, greatly weakens the resistance of this mucosa, and in the presence of large volumes of acid, and a reduction in duodenal mucosal bicarbonate production,[86] ulcers develop.

Management of Dyspepsia

Gastroenterologists in the UK follow the recent guidelines issued by the British Society of Gastroenterology. These were produced by a specially convened working group that updated its report in April 2002. We find them, on balance, the most appropriate guidelines to follow, although there are clear national differences dictated by regional epidemiologic factors and disease prevalences as well as differences in methods of providing national health care. The section below is largely based on the document produced by the British Society of Gastroenterology.

Investigations
- It is advisable that waiting times for investigation should not exceed 4 weeks, and ideally investigations should be available within 2 weeks. This clearly is particularly important if alarm symptoms are present.
- The best investigation for uncomplicated dyspepsia is endoscopy.
- A rapid urease slide test (e.g. CLO) should be checked at endoscopy in all patients in whom the *H. pylori* status is not already known. We believe this applies equally in the presence or absence of endoscopic abnormalities. In *H. pylori*-negative patients with suspected NSAID and aspirin gastropathy, Crohn's disease, lymphoma and other unusual causes of ulceration as discussed previously, biopsy of the lesions is also necessary.

In which dyspeptic patients is diagnostic endoscopy appropriate?
- Any dyspeptic patient with alarm symptoms or signs (see page 21).
- Any patient over the age of 55 with recent (<1 year) onset dyspepsia of at least 4 weeks duration.

In which dyspeptic patients is endoscopy inappropriate?

- Patients with documented duodenal ulcer disease who have responded to treatment symptomatically.
- Patients under 55 with uncomplicated dyspepsia.
- Patients who have recently undergone a satisfactory endoscopy for the same symptoms.

Treatment before investigation: is it acceptable?

Yes, provided patients are under 55, symptoms are troublesome enough and there are no alarm symptoms. If this course is to be followed, it is recommended that *H.pylori* testing be undertaken, while endoscopy is not recommended in such patients.

Patients over 55 years of age with first onset dyspepsia **should undergo prompt endoscopy**. The guidelines suggest that antisecretory drugs should be withheld or stopped 4 weeks before endoscopy, as these may mask significant pathology at the time of endoscopy. In practice, patients are usually told to stop taking their medication 2 weeks before endoscopy, as invariably they complain of intolerable symptoms. The patients are usually asked to use antacids liberally in the event of significant recurrence of symptoms, and most adhere to advice about stopping antisecretory therapy.

Treatment post-diagnosis

Major diagnoses

In the original guidelines, the panel of experts recommended treatment of *H. pylori* infection only for duodenal and gastric ulcer. This was based on the available evidence at the time but has now been superseded by more recent trials in favour of the "Test and treat" strategy. This strategy in uncomplicated dyspepsia assumes that all cases of "undiagnosed" functional dyspepsia associated with *H. pylori* will receive eradication therapy, and thus it follows that **eradication of *H. pylori* in known cases of functional dyspepsia is an acceptable therapy**.

Duodenal ulcer

H. pylori-positive duodenal ulcer

Treat with *H. pylori* eradication therapy. It is advisable to confirm the presence of *H. pylori* infection before treatment, but since the prevalence of *H. pylori* infection is so high in DU, it may be unnecessary to do that. The recommended eradication regimens are as follows.

First Line: 1 week triple therapy (no continued antisecretory required)

PPI (standard dose twice daily) or RBC (ranitidine bismuth citrate), plus amoxycillin 500 mg–1 g twice daily or

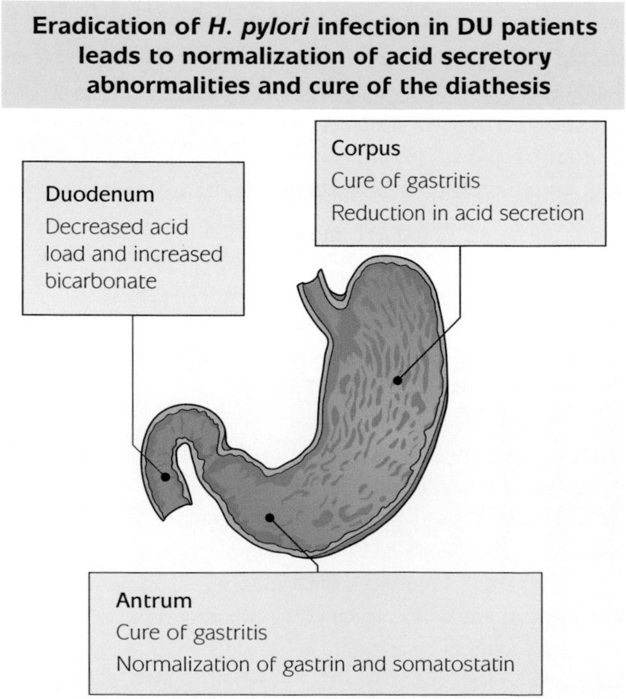

Figure 22. Eradication of *H. pylori* infection in DU patients leads to normalization of acid secretory abnormalities and cure of the diathesis.

metronidazole 400–500 mg twice daily, plus clarithromycin 500 mg twice daily (Figure 23).

It is sensible to avoid metronidazole if the patient has had a previous course of treatment with this agent as the likelihood of resistance is very high.

Second line: quadruple therapy

PPI (standard dose twice daily), plus bismuth subcitrate 120 mg four times daily, plus metronidazole 400–500 mg three times daily, plus tetracycline 500 mg four times daily (Figure 23).

Follow-up

Asymptomatic patients: Repeat endoscopy is not needed. A UBT (ideally ^{13}C) should be performed in all patients (1 month or longer after the end of *H. pylori* eradication treatment) if symptoms persist or recur. A UBT is also required in any patient

---

Treatment of *H. pylori* infection

How to treat *H. pylori* infection

First line therapy

PPI (RBC) standard dose bid
+ clarithromycin 500 mg bid (C)
+ amoxycillin 1000 mg bid (A)
or metronidazole 500 mg bid (M)*
for a minimum of 7 days
*CA is preferred to CM as it may favour best results
with second line PPI quadruple therapy

In case of failure

Second line therapy

PPI standard dose + bismuth subsalicylate/
subcitrate 120 mg qid + metronidazole 500 mg tid
+ tetracycline 500 mg qid for a minimum of 7 days
If bismuth is not available, PPI-based triple
therapy should be used

Figure 23. Treatment of *H. pylori* infection.

whose ulcer had presented with complications and who would otherwise be given long-term anti-secretory treatment to prevent recurrence. If the result of the breath test is negative, we recommend no further treatment. If the result is positive, a second course of eradication therapy should be prescribed as discussed in the section on complicated peptic ulcers. Assessment of antibiotic sensitivity may be considered in those with persistent *H. pylori* although most units are not equipped or do not have the resources to do sensitivity testing on a routine basis.

Symptomatic after initial symptom response: A UBT is indicated. If negative, clinical re-evaluation is necessary and if positive, repeat anti-*H. pylori* treatment.

H. pylori-negative duodenal ulcer
Antisecretory therapy
Cimetidine 800mg nocte (nightly) is cheapest. GI referral is advised if ulcers are not associated with NSAID therapy. NSAIDs should be stopped if possible and if symptoms persist patients may need specialist GI review.

Long-term antisecretory drugs
Low dose PPI "maintenance" is required only in patients with persistent *H. pylori* infection or those at risk of serious complications while receiving NSAIDs. NICE guidance on cyclo-oxygenase-2-specific antagonists should be considered in these instances.

Erosive duodenitis
Erosive duodenitis is regarded as part of the spectrum of the *H. pylori*-induced DU diathesis and as such behaves physiologically in a similar fashion. *H. pylori* eradication is therefore indicated in this condition.

Gastric ulcer
H. pylori is present in about 70% of GU cases and most of the remainder are associated with NSAIDs. Cytological smears and biopsies should be taken for histology and a urease test should be performed at endoscopy.

H. pylori-positive gastric ulcer

Anti-*H.pylori* therapy as for DU, followed by antisecretory therapy for two months. The reason for this latter recommendation is the lack of evidence that GUs heal as quickly as DUs after *H. pylori* eradication alone. Long-term treatment with a PPI or misoprostol should be considered in patients with proven ulcer who *continue* to take NSAIDs.

H. pylori-negative gastric ulcer

Standard antisecretory therapy for 2 months. NSAIDs should be stopped if possible. Full dose PPI is more effective than H_2 antagonist if NSAID is continued. Long-term treatment with misoprostol *or PPI* should be considered in patients with proven ulcer who cannot stop the NSAID.

Follow up of all cases of gastric ulcer

Repeat endoscopy with biopsies is essential until the ulcer is completely healed because of the small risk that a cancer is present. As discussed previously, this risk may have been overblown, but it is wise to adhere to this cautious approach. If the ulcer remains unhealed for 6 months, then surgery should be considered, if the patient is medically fit.

Oesophagitis

H. pylori infection is not associated with this condition, and in fact there is evidence to suggest that infection with virulent *H. pylori* strains may protect against severe complications of GORD. Patients should be informed of the key relationship between obesity and reflux symptoms, particularly heartburn. Weight loss is believed to be effective treatment in some patients, but the evidence for this is anecdotal. Propping up the head of the bed (by 6 inches) has been shown to be beneficial in some studies, and patients should be advised to avoid factors that provoke symptoms including bending, alcoholic beverages and fatty foods.

Treatment is usually very successful and a 4-week course is a reasonable initial attempt. There is no doubt that PPIs are superior to other forms of therapy, but many patients obtain adequate symptom control from antacids, raft preparations, H_2 antagonists or prokinetic agents. Whatever therapy is chosen, an attempt should always be made to titrate to the agent that provides symptomatic relief at the lowest dose and, by inference, the lowest cost.

Follow up

Repeat endoscopy is not justifiable except to check for healing of oesophageal ulcers, dilatation of strictures, or when anaemia that is believed to be secondary to oesophagitis fails to resolve on treatment. The impact of endoscopic surveillance on the long-term management and outcome of Barrett's oesophagus remains controversial and awaits long-term follow-up studies. Some patients may need longer term treatment to maintain symptom relief. However, such prescriptions should be reviewed and attempts to titrate the dose against symptom relief, or to switch to cheaper remedies, should be made regularly.

Functional dyspepsia

This has already been discussed in detail in previous sections.

Lifestyle advice relevant to all dyspeptic disease

There is insufficient evidence to recommend any particular lifestyle advice. Smokers should be advised not to smoke for obvious general health reasons, and healthy eating should be encouraged, though neither are known to affect these symptoms. Figures 24 and 25 relate to patient information sheets for dyspepsia that we frequently use and are provided courtesy of the GI Unit in Aberdeen Royal Infirmary.

Other guidelines for the management of dyspepsia

For the sake of completeness, we have provided in this section the so-called Maastricht Guidelines for management of *H. pylori* infection (Tables 11, 12 and 13). These were the product of years of experience in the *H. pylori* field within the European Union. This expertise culminated in two consensus meetings both held in

Patient information sheets
Lifestyle advice: Indigestion

Some useful tips on how to reduce symptoms of indigestion

- **Try to eat regular meals at regular intervals**
  This prevents build up of acid within the stomach

- **Antacids are best taken when symptoms occur or are expected, usually between meals and at bedtime**

- **Avoid dietary items that cause you indigestion**
  Hot curries and fatty foods are particularly bad

- **Avoid large meals in the evening**
  They are especially bad for causing indigestion

- **Avoid using anti-inflammatory painkillers such as ibuprofen (nurofen, brufen), aspirin or medicines containing aspirin**
  These drugs can irritate the stomach lining. Paracetamol would be a suitable alternative painkiller. If you think a drug is causing symptoms, mention it to your doctor.

- **Try to lose weight if you are overweight**

- **STOP SMOKING!**
  Smoking weakens the lining of the stomach against acid and can delay healing of ulcers

- **Try not to exceed the maximum recommended level of alcohol per week**
  Alcohol relaxes the valve between gullet and stomach and makes acid reflux easier. Binge drinking is particularly harmful.
  Recommended maximum weekly intake is 21 units for females and 30 units for males. (One unit = half a pint = glass of wine = measure of spirits)

Figure 24. Patient information sheets. Lifestyle advice: Indigestion.

Patient information sheets
Lifestyle advice: Heartburn/reflux

Heartburn is a sharp burning pain in the centre of the chest caused when acid refluxes up from the stomach into the gullet.

Some useful tips on how to reduce symptoms of heartburn/reflux

- **Avoid tight clothing**
  The pressure on the abdomen tends to make reflux worse.

- **Avoid stooping or bending especially after eating**

- **Avoid eating just before going to bed**

- **Try losing some weight**

- **If you smoke, try to stop or reduce smoking**
  Smoking decreases the pressure in the valve between the gullet and the stomach. This means acid can reflux out of the stomach into the gullet much more readily. Smoking also decreases salivation and the stomach's resistance to acid attack.

- **Try avoiding food items and drinks that cause symptoms**
  Fat, chocolate, tea, coffee, alcohol, citrus fruits, tomatoes and spicy foods may cause reflux by relaxing the valve between the gullet and stomach in the same way as smoking.

- **Try chewing gum**
  This increases production of saliva, which can help to wash acid out of the gullet.

- **Raise the head of the bed**
  Use blocks of wood or bricks to raise the head of the bed by 8 inches (increasing the number or size of pillows is not effective). This is very effective in preventing acid reflux overnight and in encouraging healing of the lining of the gullet.

Figure 25. Patient information sheets. Lifestyle advice: Heartburn/reflux.

Maastricht, Netherlands. Maastricht II guidelines were published in 2002, and to a great extent reflect current practices within the European Union. There are clear differences between these and current practices in North America, which are discussed in a separate section below. Table 11 outlines the management strategies in primary care, a special aspect of the Maastricht Guidelines that recognised the key role played by primary care physicians. Table 12 outlines the recommended indications for *H. pylori* eradication, the level of the recommendation and the supporting evidence. Table 13 outlines the strongly recommended indications for *H. pylori* eradication therapy and the strength of supporting evidence. Finally,

Key management strategies in primary care

- A "test and treat" approach should be used in adult patients under the age of 45 years (the age cut-off may vary locally) with persistent dyspepsia, having excluded those with predominantly GORD symptoms, NSAID users and patients with alarm symptoms.

- Diagnosis of infection should be by urea breath test or stool antigen test.

- Always test for successful eradication, by urea breath test or endoscopy-based test if endoscopy is clinically indicated.

- Stool antigen test is the alternative if urea breath test is not available.

- In uncomplicated duodenal ulcer patients, eradication therapy does not need to be followed by further antisecretory treatment.

- A "search and treat" strategy is recommended for peptic ulcer patients on long-term and intermittent antisecretory therapy.

Table 11. Summary of the key management strategies for *Helicobacter pylori* infection in primary care. Reproduced with permission from Malfertheiner P *et al.*; The European *Helicobacter Pylori* Study Group (EHPSG).Current concepts in the management of *Helicobacter pylori* infection—the Maastricht 2-2000 Consensus Report. *Aliment Pharmacol Ther* 2002; **16:** 167–180.

Recommended indications for *Helicobacter pylori* eradication therapy, and related statements, in further disease areas, the level of the recommendation and the strength of the supporting evidence

Disease area	Level of recommendation or statement	Strength of supporting evidence
H. pylori-positive functional dyspepsia		
H. pylori eradication is an appropriate option.	Advisable	2
This leads to long-term symptom improvement in a subset of patients.	Strong	2
GORD		
H. pylori eradication:		
Is not associated with GORD development in most cases.	Strong	3
Does not exacerbate existing GORD.	Advisable	3
H. pylori should be eradicated, though in patients requiring long-term profound acid suppression.	Advisable	3
NSAIDs		
H. pylori eradication:		
Reduces the incidence of ulcer given prior to NSAID use.	Advisable	2
Alone is insufficient to prevent recurrent ulcer bleeding in high-risk NSAID users.	Strong	2
Does not enhance healing of gastric or duodenal ulcers in patients receiving antisecretory therapy who continue to take NSAIDs.	Strong	1
H. pylori and NSAIDs/aspirin are independent risk factors for peptic ulcer disease	Advisable	2

Table 12. Recommended indications for *Helicobacter pylori* eradication therapy, and related statements, in further disease areas, the level of the recommendation and the strength of the supporting evidence. Reproduced with permission from Malfertheiner P *et al.*, The European *Helicobacter Pylori* Study Group (EHPSG). Current concepts in the management of *Helicobacter pylori* infection—the Maastricht 2-2000 Consensus Report. *Aliment Pharmacol Ther* 2002; **16:** 167–180.

Strongly recommended indications for *Helicobacter pylori* eradication therapy and the strength of the supporting evidence	
Indication (*H. pylori*-positive)	**Strength of supporting evidence**
Peptic ulcer disease (active or not, including complicated ulcer)	1
MALToma	2
Atrophic gastritis	2
Post-gastric cancer resection	3
Patients who are first-degree relatives of gastric cancer patients	3
Patients' wishes (after full consultation with their physician)	4

MALToma = mucosa-associated lymphoid tissue lymphoma

Table 13. Strongly recommended indications for *Helicobacter pylori* eradication therapy and the strength of the supporting evidence. Reproduced with permission from Malfertheiner P *et al.*, The European *Helicobacter Pylori* Study Group (EHPSG). Current concepts in the management of *Helicobacter pylori* infection—the Maastricht 2-2000 Consensus Report. *Aliment Pharmacol Ther* 2002; **16:** 167–180.

Characteristics of *Helicobacter pylori* infection in elderly subjects compared to young or adult subjects

Prevalence of infection	• Increases with age in asymptomatic subjects. • Decreases in elderly subjects with PUD (50–70% versus 80–90% of adult peptic ulcer patients. • Higher in elderly subjects who have lived in nursing homes for longer times. • No significant correlation between *H. pylori* infection and cognitive status, disability, nutritional status and extracardiac atherosclerosis.
Indications for eradication	• Similar benefit of curing *H. pylori* infection in young and elderly patients with peptic ulcer, gastric MALT lymphoma, non-ulcer dyspepsia, chronic atrophic gastritis. • In elderly subjects, eradication therapy alone is not sufficient to prevent peptic ulcer or re-bleeding related to acute or chronic NSAID use. • No definite role of *H. pylori* eradication in elderly users of low-dose aspirin as well as in elderly patients with GORD.
Diagnosis of infection	• Test-and-treatment strategies are not useful and may be unsafe in elderly subjects. • Rapid urease test and histology may have lower sensitivity in the elderly than in adults. • In the elderly, a second test for *H. pylori* should be performed if a urease-based or histological test is negative.
Post-treatment evaluation	• ^{13}C-urea breath test has higher sensitivity and specificity than serology and is unaffected by cognitive function, disability, co-morbidity and co-treatments. • The potential role of stool antigen test remains to be explored in old age.
Treatment	• One-week, PPI-based triple therapies are very effective in elderly patients. • Low doses of both PPIs and clarithromycin (in combination with amoxicillin or nitroimidazoles) are sufficient to obtain excellent cure rates in elderly patients. • Concomitant diseases and concomitant treatments did not influence the efficacy of anti-*H. pylori* therapy. • Similar to young and adults, low compliance and antibiotic resistance are the main factors related to treatment failure.

PUD = peptic ulcer disease; GORD = gastro-oesophageal reflux disease; MALT = mucosa-associated lymphoid tissue; NSAID = non-steroidal anti-inflammatory drug; PPI = proton pump inhibitor.

Table 14. Characteristics of *Helicobacter pylori* infection in elderly subjects compared with young or adult subjects.[85]

Table 14 outlines the primary characteristics and management of *H. pylori* infection in the elderly compared with young or adult subjects.[87] These were not part of the Maastricht guidelines but we include them here for their own very important contribution.

Management of dyspepsia in the USA

The management of dyspepsia by generalists in the USA is very similar to that in other Western countries, including Europe and Australia. Generally, patients with dyspepsia lasting more than 4 weeks in duration and who are less than 45–50 years old undergo a clinical evaluation and, if no alarm symptoms are present, a non-invasive test for *H. pylori* is performed. If positive, patients are given eradication therapy and followed up. If patients are *H. pylori*-negative or if treatment of *H. pylori* fails to improve their symptoms, they are then given acid-suppression (usually PPI) for 4–8 weeks. If this fails, they are then either switched to another acid-suppressive regimen or taken to endoscopy. If an organic cause for dyspepsia is found at endoscopy, then specific management is initiated. If patients are diagnosed with functional dyspepsia, they are clinically re-evaluated, and treated with other medications that have only marginal benefit, such as tricyclic anti-depressants, antispasmodics, simethicone, etc. Close follow up with reassurance is the cornerstone of management of these patients.

Proton pump inhibitors

In view of the major role played by proton pump inhibitors (PPIs) in the management of dyspepsia, we have dedicated an exclusive section to address this class of drug. This section is not meant to be either comprehensive or promotional, but simply outlines aspects of some of the world's most commonly prescribed drugs.

The gastric proton pump H^+, K^+-ATPase, is an enzyme that is composed of two subunits, a larger α catalytic subunit and a smaller β glycosylated subunit. The enzyme transports H^+ outward in exchange for uptake of K^+, and is able to generate a concentration of approximately 160 mmol/L H^+. This corresponds to a pH of 0.80. In the unstimulated parietal cell, the proton pump is present in cytoplasmic tubules and does not generate acid.

Once stimulated, the pumps get exposed in the microvilli of the parietal cell canaliculus, and a K^+, Cl^- pathway is activated.

PPIs began their development in the mid-1970s in Sweden with work on a failed antiviral agent that was later modified to timoprazole. Further modifications resulted in the synthesis of omeprazole, the first of the PPIs to reach the market. The drug was launched in 1988 at the Rome World Congress of Gastroenterology. The basic molecular structure of omeprazole, a substituted benzimidazole, has formed the basis of all other PPIs that have been introduced to the market thus far (lansoprazole, pantoprazole and rabeprazole). The latest addition is esomeprazole, which is the S-isomer of omeprazole. In addition to sharing the core structure, these compounds generally have similar properties. They are all ampholytic weak bases and accumulate as prodrugs in the canaliculus of the active parietal cell. The prodrugs are activated by acid to form the reactive sulfenamide derivative. These then react by creating disulphide bonds with one or more exposed cysteine residues on the luminal surface of the enzyme. Recovery of gastric pump activity after inhibition with PPIs is due to both reversal of binding by disulphide-reducing agents and to pump synthesis.[88]

PPIs work maximally when acid secretion is stimulated. This explains why the drugs are given before or at the first meal of the day, usually with once-daily dosing. If more rapid acid inhibition is desired, twice-daily dosing is considered. H_2 antagonists should not be co-administered with PPIs and in fact can lead to marked reduction in efficacy. If clinically indicated, they could be given at night with the PPI given in the morning, to ensure maximal efficacy. Generally, it takes at least 3 days for steady-state inhibition of stimulated acid output to be achieved by PPIs. The lag is due to the maximal number of pumps active during the so-called dwell time of the drug in blood. To improve the response to acid inhibition in the initial phase of treatment, it is more sensible to divide the dose rather than increase it.

The PPIs have made a major impact on gastrointestinal practice since they were introduced in the late 1980s. They have become established as the mainstay of treatment for GORD and also as indispensable constituents of *H. pylori* eradication regimes. They are used to treat *H. pylori*-negative peptic ulcers, NSAID-induced ulcers and as maintenance against healed ulcers that had bled. However, the majority of patients who are prescribed PPIs fall into the categories of uninvestigated dyspepsia or functional dyspepsia. Naturally, as the dyspepsia market is global and is huge, there is tremendous competition between the different pharmaceutical companies. Due to the sheer volume of the available literature, it is often very difficult for specialists and non-specialists alike to handle critically this scientific and marketing information. In our humble opinion, all five PPIs are very effective and perform admirably in the indicated clinical situations. The majority of practitioners share this opinion, and indeed any subtle differences between the PPIs are often of academic interest. We would be happy to use any of them interchangeably for the majority of the clinical indications.

In the UK's hospital and general practice, the decision to use a particular PPI is often dictated by the agreed medicines policy of the Health Board. Certain drugs make it onto the Board's Drug Formulary based largely on local considerations. For example, a pharmaceutical company may negotiate a much more attractive deal with a particular Health Board that the decision becomes purely economic. In the absence of any major differences between the main PPIs, this approach could be morally justified. There is clearly a huge pressure on GPs to reduce the PPI budget. In 1998, the NHS in England and Wales spent £314m on PPIs. The National Institute for Clinical Excellence (NICE) estimated that if GPs were more circumspect in their use of PPIs, the NHS could save £50m ($75m) a year.[89] The NICE document provides guidance that allows for the reduction of unnecessary PPI usage, and we recommend consultation with this document (www.nice.org.uk).

Are there any considerations that differentiate between the five available PPIs?

- **Licensed indications:** all PPIs are licensed for the major dyspeptic indications, including GORD healing and maintenance, DU, GU, and *H. pylori* eradication. Understandably, the older PPIs (omeprazole and lansoprazole) have wider licensed indications by virtue of having been available for much longer. The more recent PPIs will in due course gain licenses for NSAID-related ulcer healing, maintenance after healing, and prophylaxis. Omeprazole is the only PPI licensed for dual eradication therapy, but since this is a discredited regime in most countries, this offers no particular advantage.

- **Bioavailability:** there is no doubt that esomeprazole (the S-isomer) is more potent than omeprazole (the R-isomer). Studies indicate that esomeprazole has higher and more consistent bioavailability than omeprazole, which results in a greater area under the plasma concentration–time curve.[90] Consequently, more of the drug reaches the parietal cell and there is more inhibition of gastric acid secretion. It has been estimated that esomeprazole is four times more potent than omeprazole. It is no surprise therefore that studies comparing esomeprazole 40mg with omeprazole 20mg and 40mg found the S-isomer more potent and efficacious. This superior pharmacological efficacy has also been shown in some studies comparing esomeprazole with other PPIs.[90] It remains unclear, however, if equivalent doses have been compared in these studies.

- **Duration of acid inhibition:** the half-lives of recovery of acid secretion for the different PPIs in humans were found to be as follows: lansoprazole less than 15h, omeprazole and rabeprazole less than 30h, while for pantoprazole the half-life was approximately 46h. The recovery of gastric pump activity after treatment with omeprazole, esomeprazole, lansoprazole, and rabeprazole is due both to reversal of binding by disulphide-reducing agents and to new pump synthesis. However, for pantoprazole, recovery is mainly due to new pump synthesis, and this profile is probably related to the unique binding of pantoprazole to cysteine 822, a binding site that is buried deep within the membrane domain of the pump and may therefore be inaccessible to reducing agents.[88] These interesting observations suggest but do not prove that prolonged binding of pantoprazole may confer a longer duration of action in comparison with other PPIs. The clinical significance of this remains to be established.

- **Hepatic metabolism:** all the PPIs, except rabeprazole, are metabolised primarily by the hepatic cytochrome P450 enzyme system. This system is polymorphic, and indeed common genetic polymorphisms of the *CYP*2C19 iso-enzyme affect the clearance and bioavailability of PPIs. This can lead to inconsistency in terms of acid suppression and clinical efficacy across the *CYP*2C19 genotypes for all PPIs except for rabeprazole.[91] However, these genetic polymorphisms seem to be common only in Asian populations and do not seem to have a major impact in Caucasian populations. It is very likely, however, that other genetic polymorphisms that are relevant to Caucasians will be uncovered in the near future, and this would help explain the clinical heterogeneity seen in response to PPI therapy. Interestingly, omeprazole and, more markedly, esomeprazole differ from the other PPIs in that their bioavailability increases over the first week of treatment. These two PPIs progressively reduce their hepatic clearance with repeat dosing by virtue of impairing the activity of hepatic CYP2C19.[91]

- **Efficacy in PPI-based triple therapy for the eradication of *H. pylori* infection:** adequate data is available from randomised controlled trials comparing the efficacy of omeprazole, lansoprazole, pantoprazole, and rabeprazole in PPI-based triple therapy. Review of the literature indicates that the use of lansoprazole, omeprazole, or pantoprazole combined with two antibiotics yields similar high eradication rates.[92] Similar data is available for rabeprazole.[93]

- **Side effect profile:** all PPIs have a very safe side effect profile, and there have been no major problems reported with any of them. However, one must remember that these drugs have only been available for a relatively short time, and their wide prescription has only occurred in the past 10 years. Generally, there are no major differences among the five PPIs in relation to specific side effects. Clinical experience indicates, however, that a side effect with one (e.g. headache or skin rash) may not necessarily occur with another, and it is certainly worth trying a change in PPI before giving up on this class of drug.

- **Interaction with other drugs:** most experience is understandably with the older PPIs (omeprazole and lansoprazole). Omeprazole is thought to enhance the effects of warfarin and phenytoin, whereas interaction with lansoprazole possibly differs. This may favour use of lansoprazole in epileptics or those requiring anticoagulation. Lansoprazole possibly accelerates metabolism of oral contraceptives.

- **Clinical experience with the PPIs:** the medical profession is quite appropriately conservative when it comes to changing prescribing habits. For this reason, many practitioners will continue to prescribe the older PPIs because they understand these drugs better (e.g. able to titrate the doses up or down without difficulty, or understand drug interactions), and because the newer drugs offer no major advantage. Only when experience with the newer drugs becomes more established, or if the cost reduction is so much more impressive, will practitioners opt for the newer members of a class of drug. The competition between the companies can only translate to benefit for patients, health care providers, and health care planners.

- **Formulations of the drugs:** at present, omeprazole and pantoprazole are the only PPIs available as intravenous preparations. Another situation where formulation is very important is in patients who cannot ingest tablets or capsules. Omeprazole is available as a dispersible tablet, and lansoprazole is available as a suspension.

- **Cost:** as mentioned above, this often varies from one region to another, but, generally, lansoprazole, rabeprazole and pantoprazole are cheaper than omeprazole and esomeprazole. The first three have very similar prices.

Future Developments

There is no doubt that the discovery of *H. pylori* has created a revolution in gastroenterology, and dyspeptic diseases have benefited the most from this revolution. Troublesome duodenal ulcers requiring protracted medical therapy are now easily cured with a 1-week course of antibiotics. Unphysiological and potentially disastrous surgical procedures are now rightly confined to the history books.

However, we still have some major questions to address before declaring victory on ulcer disease. For a start, the proportion of non-*H. pylori* peptic ulcers seems to be growing. This may be a reflection of the increased use of NSAIDs in an ever-ageing population, but there is an impression that we are seeing more of the so-called CLO negative ulcers, even in younger subjects. The use of NSAIDs is likely to increase dramatically in the next 10 years, especially when their protective effects against cancers of all sorts are fully appreciated. As such, we should double our efforts to understand how these ulcers form and how to prevent them.

The best antibiotic therapy against *H. pylori* is still based on a cocktail of three drugs and, as yet, we have no "magic bullet" to cure this infection. The publication of the full genome of *H. pylori* in 1997 has increased exponentially the search for novel mechanisms of attack against the organism. It is likely that a single antibiotic agent with a novel mechanism of action will be discovered in the next decade. This will certainly be very lucrative for whichever drug company handles the discovery. This is particularly pertinent because efforts to develop a therapeutic or prophylactic vaccine have met with disappointing results so far. The desire or appropriateness to vaccinate large populations is also shrouded in scientific doubt.

There remains great uncertainty regarding the best management of functional dyspepsia. This failure stems from our lack of understanding of the pathophysiology of this disease. The stimulus to understand the pathogenesis is subdued by the non-serious nature of the condition (although it causes considerable morbidity) and the availability of expensive medications that have traditionally kept the lid over this condition. There has been some growth in research focusing on visceral sensitivity and visceral reflexes, with a suggestion that at least some patients with functional gut disorders have altered visceral perception. This has opened the way for trials of drugs that modulate visceral sensitivity in this condition.

The most exciting development stems from the realization that *H. pylori* infection could act as a paradigm for gene–environment interactions in human disease. The appreciation that a microbial agent interacting with host genetic factors could lead to divergent clinical outcomes will open the way to understanding more complex human diseases such as cancer and chronic inflammatory conditions.

Frequently Asked Questions

What is the best treatment regime for *H. pylori* infection?
First line therapy for *H. pylori* consists of either a proton pump inhibitor (PPI) twice a day (e.g. omeprazole 20 mg bid) OR ranitidine-bismuth citrate (RBC) twice a day (400 mg bid) AND amoxicillin (1000 mg qd or bid) OR metronidazole (500 mg bid) AND clarithromycin (500 mg bid), for at least 10 days. If this regimen fails to eradicate the bacterium, quadruple therapy should be initiated, which consists of a PPI bid, bismuth subsalicylate (525 mg qid), tetracycline (500 mg qid) and metronidazole (500 mg tid), for 14 days.

What happens if antibiotics fail to eradicate *H. pylori*?
Although successful eradication of *H. pylori* requires multiple medications, the absolute failure rate for treating the infection is very low, in part, due to the multiplicity of treatment regimens available. For example, quadruple therapy achieves cure rates of approximately 90% in patients who have failed at least 2 previous therapies and who are colonized with metronidazole- and clarithromycin-resistant strains.

Why do I have to take a cocktail of drugs to kill *H. pylori*?
The stomach presents unique barriers to antibiotic efficacy that are usually not encountered within other anatomic niches of the human body. These include an acidic pH, peristalsis, active secretion, and a semi-permeable mucous barrier overlying the epithelium. Some antibiotics are less effective at lower pH (e.g. amoxycillin, clarithromycin) while other antibiotics (e.g. metronidazole) rapidly induce resistance in *H. pylori* strains, which decreases therapeutic efficacy. Many antibiotics exert only minimal bacteriostatic or bactericidal effects. Therefore, elimination of *H. pylori* requires multiple drugs for prolonged durations (7–14 days) to overcome these obstacles.

How fast will my symptoms settle?

This is completely dependent on the underlying clinical lesion. If your symptoms are due to peptic ulcer disease, treatment of *H. pylori* and acid suppression should rapidly induce symptomatic relief. If your symptoms are secondary to non-ulcer dyspepsia, eradication of *H. pylori* is very unlikely to provide symptomatic benefit. Finally, in a subset of patients, treatment of *H. pylori* is associated with an increase in gastro-oesophageal reflux symptoms. Thus, it is difficult to predict the tempo of symptom relief without knowledge of the inciting lesion.

Will my ulcer or *H. pylori* come back if the infection is treated successfully?

The re-infection rate for *H. pylori* following successful treatment in developed countries is <0.3% per year. Therefore, it is very unlikely that you will become re-infected. However, if you ingest medications, such as aspirin or other non-steroidal anti-inflammatory medications (NSAIDs), that cause ulcers, or develop another condition such as Crohn's disease that causes ulcers, a recurrence of this lesion may develop.

Is stomach cancer hereditary?

Although most gastric cancers occur sporadically without any evidence of an inherited cancer predisposition, a small fraction of gastric cancers (1–3%) arise as the result of clearly identified inherited gastric cancer predisposition syndromes. These syndromes include two recently well-described inherited conditions, hereditary diffuse gastric cancer syndrome and hereditary nonpolyposis colon cancer syndrome, as well as Peutz–Jeghers syndrome, Cowden's syndrome, and some kindreds affected with Li–Fraumeni syndrome and familial adenomatous polyposis. Hereditary diffuse gastric cancer (HDGC) is an autosomal dominantly-inherited gastric cancer susceptibility syndrome caused by germline mutations in *CDH1*, the gene encoding E-cadherin. It is currently unclear as to whether *H. pylori* infection contributes to these types of gastric cancer.

Do my children need to undergo *H. pylori* testing?

Several studies have indicated that maternal-to-child transmission occurs at a much higher frequency than paternal-to-child transmission. However, this does not occur in every situation, so it is currently not recommended that offspring of infected patients be routinely tested for the presence of *H. pylori*.

Is *H. pylori* transmitted through sexual contact?

There is no conclusive evidence that transmission of *H. pylori* occurs via this route.[94,95] Theoretically, *H. pylori* may be transmitted sexually, during the act of oral–anal intercourse,[96] but there is no direct proof that this occurs. In practical terms, it is not necessary to eradicate the infection in spouses/partners of treated patients for fear of re-infection. A recent study by Gisbert *et al.* found that the strains in re-infected patients and their partners were different, suggesting that the patient's partner does not act as a reservoir for *H. pylori* re-infection.[97]

Do I need an endoscopy to check for *H. pylori* infection and what is the best test for ascertaining the presence of this bacterium?

Several techniques can be used to diagnose *H. pylori,* and these can be classified as either invasive or non-invasive. Invasive methods require endoscopy with biopsy and include histological techniques, rapid urease tests, culture, or polymerase chain reaction. Non-invasive tests include urea breath tests, which detect $^{13}CO_2$ or $^{14}CO_2$ in expired breath samples following ingestion of labelled urea. High values signify the presence of gastric urease activity, which is nearly always due to the presence of *H. pylori*. Another non-invasive test is serologic detection of *H. pylori* which is based on measuring anti-*H. pylori* antibodies. Finally, the *H. pylori* stool antigen test can detect the presence of *H. pylori*-specific proteins in faeces. Although none of the currently available diagnostic tests are completely reliable due to differences in bacterial colonization density, many possess sufficiently high levels of accuracy so as to permit their wide-spread and singular use, either for initial diagnosis and/or confirmation of cure.

I put on a considerable amount of weight since my ulcer was cured with eradication therapy; why is that?

There is no doubt that cured ulcer patients have an improved appetite and a general feeling of wellbeing, which lead to increased caloric intake and weight gain. There is also the recent finding that eradication of *H. pylori* infection is associated with reduced gastric expression and release of a protein called leptin. This is the protein product of the obese gene expressed primarily by adipocytes. It provides feedback information on the size of energy stores to central receptors controlling food intake, energy expenditure and body weight homeostasis. Improvements in the gastritis is associated with reduced expression of leptin and consequently weight gain.[98,99]

Do I need to be on acid inhibitory therapy for life if I had a bleeding ulcer?

This depends on whether the ulcer was caused by *H. pylori* alone or was also associated with NSAID therapy. If it was an *H. pylori* ulcer that bled, then eradication therapy followed by 6 weeks of acid inhibitory therapy should be sufficient. Confirmation of eradication of the infection is essential, and if done all therapy could stop. If the patient was also receiving NSAID therapy, then eradication of *H. pylori* will not remove the risk of further ulceration and bleeding, and the patient's need for NSAID has to be reviewed. If NSAIDs are essential, then the stomach has to be protected by either acid inhibitors or cytoprotective agents as long as the NSAIDs are required. If NSAIDs are no longer required, then further protective agents are not needed.

Is the radioactivity of the ^{14}C-urea breath test dangerous?

The degree of radioactivity in the ^{14}C-urea breath test is very small and is a fraction of what we get from a standard chest X-ray. In most people, the radioactivity is not a consideration. However, this test is not carried out on pregnant women and children and an alternative such as the non-radioactive ^{13}C-urea breath test is considered.

I was found to have *H. pylori* infection but I do not have any stomach problems; do I need to get rid of it?

This is difficult and troubling question since the vast majority of colonized persons (85%) will develop no symptoms secondary to the presence of *H. pylori* in the stomach. However, because *H. pylori* is the strongest known risk factor for gastric cancer and ulcer disease, if a person is known to be infected, they probably should be treated to reduce the risk of developing ulcers or cancer.

H. pylori causes ulcers and cancer: why don't we just get rid of it in everyone?

Most persons infected with *H. pylori* remain asymptomatic for their entire life span. Antibiotics have side-effects, some of which can be severe, and indiscriminate use of these compounds can lead to antibiotic resistance, which directly affects eradication efficacy. The cost of testing and subsequently treating entire populations would be prohibitive. Finally, there is evidence to indicate that persons infected with certain strains of *H. pylori* may be at decreased risk for developing complications of gastro-oesophageal reflux disease. Therefore, it is not recommended at this time to test and treat all persons infected with *H. pylori*.

What is the role of vaccines in the management of *H. pylori* infection?

Although people in all geographic zones have been shown to carry the bacteria, the prevalence of *H. pylori* is higher in developing countries than in developed countries. In the USA, *H. pylori* is present in 10–15% of children under age 12 compared with 50–60% of people greater than 60 years old. The rate of acquisition of new *H. pylori* infections among adults in developed countries is less than 1% per year, and most American carriers probably acquired *H. pylori* during childhood. Over the past half-century, however, progressively fewer children have been shown to carry *H. pylori*, and this decrease accelerated following the widespread use of antibiotics. These findings indicate that the prevalence of *H.*

pylori in developed countries is decreasing, and thus in these locales, vaccination is unlikely to have any benefit. In countries where infection rates are endemic, vaccines may be useful; however, at present, vaccines have not been shown to prevent or eliminate existing *H. pylori* infections in humans. Therefore, this remains a research technique.

References

1. Bytzer P, Talley NJ. Dyspepsia. *Ann Intern Med* 2001; **134:** 815–822.

2. Westbrook JI, McIntosh JH, Talley NJ. The impact of dyspepsia definition on prevalence estimates: considerations for future researchers. *Scand J Gastroenterol* 2000; **35:** 227–233.

3. Talley NJ, Colin-Jones D, Koch KL *et al.* Functional dyspepsia: a classification with guidelines for diagnosis and management. *Gastroenterol Int* 1991; **4:** 145–160.

4. Talley NJ, Weaver AL, Tesmer DL *et al.* Lack of discriminant value of dyspepsia subgroups in patients referred for upper endoscopy. *Gastroenterology* 1993; **105:** 1378–1386.

5. Penston JG, Pounder RE. A survey of dyspepsia in Great Britain. *Aliment Pharmacol Ther* 1996; **10:** 83–89.

6. Talley NJ, Boyce P, Jones M. Identification of distinct upper and lower gastrointestinal symptom groupings in an urban population. *Gut* 1998; **42:** 690–695.

7. Agreus L, Svardsudd K, Nyren O *et al.* Irritable bowel syndrome and dyspepsia in the general population: overlap and lack of stability over time. *Gastroenterology* 1995; **109:** 671–680.

8. Talley NJ, Stanghellini V, Heading RC, Koch KL, Malagelada JR, Tytgat GN. Functional gastroduodenal disorders. *Gut* 1999; **45**(Suppl 2): II37–II42.

9. Brown C, Rees WD. Dyspepsia in general practice. *BMJ* 1990; **300:** 829–830.

10. Logan R, Delaney B. ABC of the upper gastrointestinal tract: Implications of dyspepsia for the NHS. *BMJ* 2001; **323:** 675–677.

11. Haque M, Wyeth JW, Stace NH *et al.* Prevalence, severity and associated features of gastro-oesophageal reflux and dyspepsia: a population-based study. *NZ Med J* 2000; **113:** 178–181.

12. Nyren O, Adami HO, Gustavsson S *et al.* Excess sick-listing in nonulcer dyspepsia. *J Clin Gastroenterol* 1986; **8:** 339–345.

13. Guidance on the use of proton pump inhibitors in the treatment of dyspepsia. Technology Appraisal Guidance No. 7. National Institute for Clinical Excellence, July 2000. http://www.nice.org.uk/pdf/Proton.pdf 2002.

14. Talley NJ, Haque M, Wyeth JW *et al.* Development of a new dyspepsia impact scale: the Nepean Dyspepsia Index. *Aliment Pharmacol Ther* 1999; **13:** 225–235.

15. El-Omar EM, Banerjee S, Wirz A *et al.* The Glasgow Dyspepsia Severity Score—a tool for the global measurement of dyspepsia (see comments). *Eur J Gastroenterol Hepatol* 1996; **8:** 967–971.

16. McColl K, Murray L, El-Omar E *et al.* Symptomatic benefit from eradicating Helicobacter pylori infection in patients with nonulcer dyspepsia (see comments). *New Engl J Med* 1998; **339:** 1869–1874.

17. McColl KE, El Nujumi A, Murray LS *et al.* Assessment of symptomatic response as predictor of *Helicobacter pylori* status following eradication therapy in patients with ulcer. *Gut* 1998; **42:** 618–622.

18. McColl KE, Dickson A, El Nujumi A *et al.* Symptomatic benefit 1–3 years after *H. pylori* eradication in ulcer patients: impact of gastroesophageal reflux disease. *Am J Gastroenterol* 2000; **95:** 101–105.

19. Westbrook JI, McIntosh J, Talley NJ. Factors associated with consulting medical or non-medical practitioners for dyspepsia: an australian population-based study. *Aliment Pharmacol Ther* 2000; **14:** 1581–1588.

20. Gillen D, McColl KEL. Does concern about missing malignancy justify endoscopy in uncomplicated dyspepsia in patients aged less than 55? *Am J Gastroenterol* 1999; **94:** 75–79.

21. Ofman JJ, Rabeneck L. The effectiveness of endoscopy in the management of dyspepsia: a qualitative systematic review. *Am J Med* 1999; **106:** 335–346.

22. Christie J, Shepherd NA, Codling BW *et al.* Gastric cancer below the age of 55: implications for screening patients with uncomplicated dyspepsia. *Gut* 1997; **41:** 513–517.

23. Munnangi S, Sonnenberg A. Time trends of physician visits and treatment patterns of peptic ulcer disease in the United States. *Arch Intern Med* 1997; **157:** 1489–1494.

24. Misiewicz JJ. Peptic ulceration and its correlation with symptoms. *Clin Gastroenterol* 1978; **7:** 571–582.

25. Freston JW. Review article: role of proton pump inhibitors in non-H. pylori-related ulcers. *Aliment Pharmacol Ther* 2001; **15**(Suppl 2): 2–5.

26. Peura DA. The problem of *Helicobacter pylori*-negative idiopathic ulcer disease. *Baillieres Best Pract Res Clin Gastroenterol* 2000; **14**: 109–117.

27. McColl KE, El Nujumi AM, Chittajallu RS, *et al.* A study of the pathogenesis of *Helicobacter pylori* negative chronic duodenal ulceration. *Gut* 1993; **34**: 762–768.

28. McColl KE. *Helicobacter pylori*-negative ulcer disease. *J Gastroenterol* 2000; **35**(Suppl 12): 47–50.

29. Seager JM, Hawkey CJ. ABC of the upper gastrointestinal tract: Indigestion and non-steroidal anti-inflammatory drugs. *BMJ* 2001; **323**: 1236–1239.

30. Straus WL, Ofman JJ, MacLean C *et al.* Do NSAIDs cause dyspepsia? A meta-analysis evaluating alternative dyspepsia definitions. *Am J Gastroenterol* 2002; **97**: 1951–1958.

31. Wolfe MM, Lichtenstein DR, Singh G. Gastrointestinal toxicity of nonsteroidal anti-inflammatory drugs. *New Engl J Med* 1999; **340**: 1888–1899.

32. Hawkey CJ. Non-steroidal anti-inflammatory drugs and peptic ulcers. *BMJ* 1990; **300**: 278–284.

33. Henry D, Lim LL, Garcia Rodriguez LA *et al.* Variability in risk of gastrointestinal complications with individual non-steroidal anti-inflammatory drugs: results of a collaborative meta-analysis. *BMJ* 1996; **312**: 1563–1566.

34. Black RJ, Bray F, Ferlay J *et al.* Cancer incidence and mortality in the European Union: cancer registry data and estimates of national incidence for 1990. *Eur J Cancer* 1997; **33**: 1075–1107.

35. Greenlee RT, Murray T, Bolden S *et al.* Cancer statistics, 2000 CA. *Cancer J Clin* 2000; **50**(1): 7–33

36. Parkin DM, Pisani P, Ferlay J. Estimates of the worldwide incidence of 25 major cancers in 1990. *Int J Cancer* 1999; **80**: 827–841.

37. Wienbeck M, Barnert J. Epidemiology of reflux disease and reflux esophagitis. *Scand J Gastroenterol Suppl* 1989; **156**: 7–13.

38. Bainbridge ET, Nicholas SD, Newton JR *et al.* Gastro-oesophageal reflux in pregnancy. Altered function of the barrier to reflux in asymptomatic women during early pregnancy. *Scand J Gastroenterol* 1984; **19:** 85–89.

39. Bainbridge ET, Temple JG, Nicholas SP et al. Symptomatic gastro-oesophageal reflux in pregnancy. A comparative study of white Europeans and Asians in Birmingham. *Br J Clin Pract* 1983; **37:** 53–57.

40. Sonnenberg A, El Serag HB. Clinical epidemiology and natural history of gastroesophageal reflux disease. *Yale J Biol Med* 1999; **72:** 81–92.

41. Parkman HP, Fisher RS. Contributing role of motility abnormalities in the pathogenesis of gastroesophageal reflux disease. *Dig Dis* 1997; **15**(Suppl 1): 40–52.

42. Miller LS, Vinayek R, Frucht H *et al.* Reflux esophagitis in patients with Zollinger-Ellison syndrome. *Gastroenterology* 1990; **98:** 341–346.

43. Parkman HP, Harris AD, Krevsky B *et al.* Gastroduodenal motility and dysmotility: an update on techniques available for evaluation. *Am J Gastroenterol* 1995; **90:** 869–892.

44. Lundell LR, Dent J, Bennett JR *et al.* Endoscopic assessment of oesophagitis: clinical and functional correlates and further validation of the Los Angeles classification. *Gut* 1999; *45:* 172–180.

45. Kahrilas PJ, Quigley EM. Clinical esophageal pH recording: a technical review for practice guideline development. *Gastroenterology* 1996; **110:** 1982–1996.

46. Younes Z, Johnson DA. Diagnostic evaluation in gastroesophageal reflux disease. *Gastroenterol Clin North Am* 1999; **28:** 809–830.

47. Dent J, Hetzel DJ, MacKinnon MA *et al.* Evaluation of omeprazole in reflux oesophagitis. *Scand J Gastroenterol Suppl* 1989; **166:** 76–82.

48. Hetzel DJ, Dent J, Reed WD *et al.* Healing and relapse of severe peptic esophagitis after treatment with omeprazole. *Gastroenterology* 1988; **95:** 903–912.

49. Kuipers EJ, Klinkenberg-Knol EC, Meuwissen SG. Omeprazole and accelerated onset of atrophic gastritis. *Gastroenterology* 2000; **118:** 239–242.

50. Kuipers EJ, Lee A, Klinkenberg-Knol EC *et al.* Review article: the development of atrophic gastritis—*Helicobacter pylori* and the effects of acid suppressive therapy. *Aliment Pharmacol Ther* 1995; **9:** 331–340.

51. Kuipers EJ, Uyterlinde AM, Pena AS *et al.* Increase of *Helicobacter pylori*-associated corpus gastritis during acid suppressive therapy: implications for long-term safety. *Am J Gastroenterol* 1995; **90:** 1401–1406.

52. Perdikis G, Hinder RA, Lund RJ *et al.* Laparoscopic Nissen fundoplication: where do we stand? *Surg Laparosc Endosc* 1997; **7:** 17–21.

53. Talley NJ, Phung N, Kalantar JS. ABC of the upper gastrointestinal tract: Indigestion: When is it functional? *BMJ* 2001; **323:** 1294–1297.

54. El-Omar E, Penman I, Ardill JE *et al.* A substantial proportion of non-ulcer dyspepsia patients have the same abnormality of acid secretion as duodenal ulcer patients. *Gut* 1995; **36:** 534–538.

55. Fox JG. The non-*H. pylori* helicobacters: their expanding role in gastrointestinal and systemic diseases. *Gut* 2002; **50:** 273–283.

56. Everhart JE. Recent developments in the epidemiology of *Helicobacter pylori*. *Gastroenterol Clin North Am* 2000; **29:** 559–578.

57. Scott DR, Weeks D, Hong C *et al.* The role of internal urease in acid resistance of *Helicobacter pylori*. *Gastroenterology* 1998; **114:** 58–70.

58. Weeks DL, Eskandari S, Scott DR *et al.* A H+-gated urea channel: the link between *Helicobacter pylori* urease and gastric colonization. *Science* 2000; **287:** 482–485.

59. Eaton KA, Krakowka S. Effect of gastric pH on urease-dependent colonization of gnotobiotic piglets by *Helicobacter pylori*. *Infect Immun* 1994; **62:**3604–3607.

60. Tomb JF, White O, Kerlavage AR *et al.* The complete genome sequence of the gastric pathogen Helicobacter pylori. *Nature* 1997; **388:** 539–547.

61. Alm RA, Ling LS, Moir DT *et al.* Genomic-sequence comparison of two unrelated isolates of the human gastric pathogen *Helicobacter pylori*. *Nature* 1999; **397:** 176–180.

62. Keates S, Hitti YS, Upton M, Kelly CP. *Helicobacter pylori* infection activates NF-kappa B in gastric epithelial cells. *Gastroenterology* 1997; **113:** 1099–1109.

63. Keates S, Keates AC, Warny M *et al*. Differential activation of mitogen-activated protein kinases in AGS gastric epithelial cells by cag+ and cag- *Helicobacter pylori*. *J Immunol* 1999; **163**: 5552–5559.

64. Israel DA, Peek RM. Pathogenesis of *Helicobacter pylori*-induced gastric inflammation. *Aliment Pharmacol Ther* 2001; **15**: 1271–1290.

65. Peek RM, Jr., Miller GG, Tham KT *et al*. Heightened inflammatory response and cytokine expression in vivo to cagA+ *Helicobacter pylori* strains. *Lab Invest* 1995; **73**: 760–770.

66. Peek RM, Jr., Moss SF, Tham KT *et al*. *Helicobacter pylori* cagA+ strains and dissociation of gastric epithelial cell proliferation from apoptosis. *J Natl Cancer Inst* 1997; **89**: 863–868.

67. Peek RM, Jr., Wirth HP, Moss SF *et al*. *Helicobacter pylori* alters gastric epithelial cell cycle events and gastrin secretion in Mongolian gerbils. *Gastroenterology* 2000; **118**: 48–59.

68. Kuck D, Kolmerer B, Iking-Konert C *et al*. Vacuolating cytotoxin of *Helicobacter pylori* induces apoptosis in the human gastric epithelial cell line AGS. *Infect Immun* 2001; **69**: 5080–5087.

69. Peek RM, Jr., Blaser MJ. *Helicobacter pylori* and gastrointestinal tract adenocarcinomas. *Nat Rev Cancer* 2002; **2**: 28–37.

70. Logan RPH, Walker MM. ABC of the upper gastrointestinal tract: Epidemiology and diagnosis of *Helicobacter pylori* infection. *BMJ* 2001; **323**: 920–922.

71. Vaira D, Gatta L, Ricci C *et al*. Review article: diagnosis of *Helicobacter pylori* infection. *Aliment Pharmacol Ther* 2002; **16**(Suppl 1): 16–23.

72. Vakil N. Review article: the cost of diagnosing *Helicobacter pylori* infection. *Aliment Pharmacol Ther* 2001; **15**(Suppl 1): 10–15.

73. Chey WD. Accurate diagnosis of *Helicobacter pylori*. ^{14}C-urea breath test. *Gastroenterol Clin North Am* 2000; **29**: 895–902.

74. Graham DY, Klein PD. Accurate diagnosis of *Helicobacter pylori*. ^{13}C-urea breath test. *Gastroenterol Clin North Am* 2000; **29**: 885–893.

75. el Zimaity HM. Accurate diagnosis of *Helicobacter pylori* with biopsy. *Gastroenterol Clin North Am* 2000; **29:** 863–869.

76. KABIR S. Detection of *Helicobacter pylori* in faeces by culture, PCR and enzyme immunoassay. *J Med Microbiol* 2001; **50:** 1021–1029.

77. Loy CT, Irwig LM, Katelaris PH *et al.* Do commercial serological kits for *Helicobacter pylori* infection differ in accuracy? A meta-analysis. *Am J Gastroenterol* 1996; **91:** 1138–1144.

78. Stevens M, Livsey, Swann R *et al.* Evaluation of sixteen EIAs for the detection of antibodies to *Helicobacter pylori*. London: Department of Health, 1997; pp. 1–46.

79. Midolo P, Marshall BJ. Accurate diagnosis of Helicobacter pylori. Urease tests. *Gastroenterol Clin North Am* 2000; **29:** 871–878.

80. Megraud F. Advantages and disadvantages of current diagnostic tests for the detection of *Helicobacter pylori*. *Scand J Gastroenterol Suppl* 1996; **215:** 57–62.

81. Laine L, Chun D, Stein C *et al.* The influence of size or number of biopsies on rapid urease test results: a prospective evaluation. *Gastrointest Endosc* 1996; **43:** 49–53.

82. Puetz T, Vakil N, Phadnis S *et al.* The Pyloritek test and the CLO test: accuracy and incremental cost analysis. *Am J Gastroenterol* 1997; **92:** 254–257.

83. Tu TC, Lee CL, Wu CH *et al.* Comparison of invasive and noninvasive tests for detecting *Helicobacter pylori* infection in bleeding peptic ulcers. *Gastrointest Endosc* 1999; **49:** 302–306.

84. McColl KE, El-Omar E, Gillen D. *Helicobacter pylori* gastritis and gastric physiology. *Gastroenterol Clin North Am* 2000; **29:** 687–703.

85. Kuipers EJ, Lundell L, Klinkenberg-Knol EC *et al.* Atrophic gastritis and *Helicobacter pylori* infection in patients with reflux esophagitis treated with omeprazole or fundoplication. *New Engl J Med* 1996; **334:** 1018–1022.

86. Hogan DL, Rapier RC, Dreilinger A *et al.* Duodenal bicarbonate secretion: eradication of *Helicobacter pylori* and duodenal structure and function in humans. *Gastroenterology* 1996; **110:** 705–716.

87. Pilotto A, Malfertheiner P. Review article: an approach to *Helicobacter pylori* infection in the elderly. *Aliment Pharmacol Ther* 2002; **16:** 683–691.

88. Sachs G, Shin JM, Pratha V, Hogan D. Synthesis or rupture: duration of acid inhibition by proton pump inhibitors. *Drugs Today (Barc)* 2003; **39** (Suppl A): 11–14.

89. Ferriman A. NICE issues guidance for heartburn and indigestion. *BMJ* 2000; **321**(7255): 197a.

90. Lindberg P, Keeling D, Fryklund J *et al*. Review article: Esomeprazole—enhanced bio-availability, specificity for the proton pump and inhibition of acid secretion. *Aliment Pharmacol Ther* 2003; **17**(4):481–488.

91. McColl KE, Kennerley P. Proton pump inhibitors—differences emerge in hepatic metabolism. *Dig Liver Dis* 2002; **34**(7):461–467.

92. Ulmer HJ, Beckerling A, Gatz G. Recent use of proton pump inhibitor-based triple therapies for the eradication of *H. pylori*: a broad data review. *Helicobacter* 2003; **8**(2): 95–104.

93. Hawkey CJ, Atherton JC, Treichel HC, Thjodleifsson B, Ravic M. Safety and efficacy of 7-day rabeprazole- and omeprazole-based triple therapy regimens for the eradication of *Helicobacter pylori* in patients with documented peptic ulcer disease. *Aliment Pharmacol Ther* 2003; **17**(8):1065–1074.

94. Polish LB, Douglas JM, Jr., Davidson AJ *et al*. Characterization of risk factors for *Helicobacter pylori* infection among men attending a sexually transmitted disease clinic: lack of evidence for sexual transmission. *J Clin Microbiol* 1991; **29**: 2139–2143.

95. Perez-Perez GI, Witkin SS, Decker MD *et al*. Seroprevalence of *Helicobacter pylori* infection in couples. *J Clin Microbiol* 1991; **29**: 642–644.

96. Eslick GD. Sexual transmission of *Helicobacter pylori* via oral–anal intercourse. *Int J STD AIDS* 2002; **13**: 7–11.

97. Gisbert JP, Arata IG, Boixeda D *et al*. Role of partner's infection in reinfection after *Helicobacter pylori* eradication. *Eur J Gastroenterol Hepatol* 2002; **14**: 865–871.

98. Konturek JW, Konturek SJ, Kwiecien N *et al*. Leptin in the control of gastric secretion and gut hormones in humans infected with *Helicobacter pylori*. *Scand J Gastroenterol* 2001; **36**: 1148–1154.

99. Azuma T, Suto H, Ito Y *et al*. Gastric leptin and *Helicobacter pylori* infection. *Gut* 2001; **49**: 324–329.

Appendix 1 – Drugs

Drug	Trade name	Preparation	Strength	Doses used in gastrointestinal disease (adult)	Comments	Side-effects
Antacids containing aluminium and magnesium						
Aluminium hydroxide	Aludrox	Suspension	4%	5-10ml 4 times/d and nocte prn	Contraindicated in porphyria, hypophosphataemia, used to treat dyspepsia; take after meals; may impair absorption of other drugs; chew tablets before swallowing	Constipation (aluminium), laxative (magnesium)
	Alucap	Capsule	475mg	475mg 4 times/d and nocte prn		
Aluminium hydroxide + magnesium hydroxide (co-magaldrox)	Maalox TC	Tablet	600mg + 300mg	1-2 tablets or 5-10ml 4 times/d and nocte prn		
	Maalox TC	Suspension	600mg + 300mg/5ml			
	Mucogel	Suspension	220mg + 195mg/5ml	10-20ml 3 times/d and nocte prn		
Aluminium hydroxide + dimeticone + magnesium oxide	Maalox Plus	Suspension	220mg + 25mg + 195mg/5ml	5-10ml 4 times/d and nocte prn		
Aluminium hydroxide + magnesium hydroxide + oxetacaine	Mucaine	Suspension	Aluminium hydroxide susp 4.75ml + 100mg + 10mg/5ml	5-10ml 3-4 times/d and nocte prn		
Dimeticone + hydrotalcite (co-simalcite)	Altacite Plus	Suspension	125mg/500mg/5 ml	10ml between meals and nocte prn		

Antacids containing aluminium and magnesium

Drug	Trade name	Preparation	Strength	Doses used in gastrointestinal disease (adult)	Comments	Side-effects
Aluminium hydroxide/magnesium carbonate co-gel + magnesium alginate + magnesium carbonate + potassium bicarbonate	Algicon	Tablet	360mg + 500mg + 320mg + 100mg	1-2 tablets 4 times/d and nocte prn	Contraindicated in porphyria, hypophosphataemia; used to treat dyspepsia and mild symptoms of gastrointestinal reflux disease; take after meals; may impair absorption of other drugs; chew tablets before swallowing	Constipation (aluminium), laxative (magnesium)
	Algicon	Suspension	140mg + 250mg + 175mg + 50mg/5ml	10-20ml 4 times/d and nocte prn		
Alginic acid + aluminium hydroxide + magnesium trisilicate + sodium bicarbonate	Gastrocote	Tablet	200mg + 80mg + 40mg + 70mg	1-2 tablets 4 times/d and nocte prn		
Aluminium hydroxide + magnesium trisilicate + sodium alginate + sodium bicarbonate	Gastrocote	Suspension	80mg + 40mg + 220mg + 70mg/5ml	5-15ml 3-4 times/d and nocte prn		
Alginic acid + aluminium hydroxide + magnesium trisilicate + sodium bicarbonate	Gaviscon	Tablet	500mg + 100mg + 25mg + 170mg	1-2 tablets 4 times/d and nocte prn		
Sodium alginate + sodium bicarbonate + calcium carbonate	Gaviscon	Suspension	250mg + 133.5mg + 80mg/5ml	10-20ml 4 times/d and nocte prn		

Drug	Trade name	Preparation	Strength	Doses used in gastrointestinal disease (adult)	Comments	Side-effects
Antacids containing aluminium and magnesium						
Sodium alginate + potassium bicarbonate	Gaviscon Advance	Suspension	500mg + 100mg/5ml	5–10ml 4 times/d and nocte prn	Contraindicated in porphyria, hypophosphataemia; used to treat dyspepsia and mild symptoms of gastrointestinal reflux disease; take after meals; may impair absorption of other drugs; chew tablets before swallowing	Constipation (aluminium), laxative (magnesium)
Sodium bicarbonate + sodium alginate + calcium carbonate	Peptac	Suspension	133.5mg + 250mg + 80mg/5ml	10–20ml 4 times/d and nocte prn		
Calcium carbonate + magnesium carbonate + sodium alginate	Rennie Duo	Suspension	600mg + 70mg + 150mg	10ml 4 times/d and nocte prn		
H₂ receptor antagonists						
Cimetidine	Dyspamet	Suspension	200mg/5ml	Gastric and duodenal ulceration: 400mg 2 times/d for 4–8 weeks maintenance 400mg nocte: reflux oesophagitis: 400mg 4 times/d for 4–8 weeks	Caution in hepatic and renal impairment (reduce dose), pregnancy and breast feeding, elderly; treatment may mask symptoms of gastric cancer; used to treat dyspepsia due to gastric and duodenal ulceration or NSAID-associated ulceration and reflux oesophagitis	Diarrhoea and other gastrointestinal effects, altered liver function tests, headache, dizziness, rash, tiredness, alopecia
	Tagamet	Tablet	200mg, 400mg, 800mg	ulceration: 400mg 2 times/d for 4–8 weeks (max 2.4g/d), maintenance 400mg nocte: reflux		
		Syrup	200mg/5ml	oesophagitis: 400mg 4 times/d for 4–8 weeks		
Famotidine	Pepcid	Tablet	20mg, 40mg	Gastric and duodenal ulceration: 40mg nocte for 4–8 weeks, maintenance 20mg nocte; reflux oesophagitis: 20–40mg 2 times/d for 6–12 weeks, maintenance 20mg 2 times/d	Caution in hepatic and renal impairment (reduce dose), pregnancy and breast feeding; treatment may mask symptoms of gastric cancer; used to treat dyspepsia due to gastric and duodenal ulceration or NSAID-associated ulceration and reflux oesophagitis	Diarrhoea and other gastrointestinal effects, altered liver function tests, headache, dizziness, rash, tiredness

Drug	Trade name	Preparation	Strength	Doses used in gastrointestinal disease (adult)	Comments	Side-effects
H₁ receptor antagonists						
Nizatidine	Axid	Capsule	150mg, 300mg	Gastric and duodenal ulceration: 150mg 2 times/d for 4–8 weeks, maintenance 150mg nocte; reflux oesophagitis: 150–300mg 2 times/d for up to 12 weeks	Caution in hepatic and renal impairment (reduce dose); pregnancy and breast feeding; treatment may mask symptoms of gastric cancer; used to treat dyspepsia due to gastric and duodenal ulceration or NSAID-associated ulceration and reflux oesophagitis	Diarrhoea and other gastrointestinal effects, altered liver function tests, headache, dizziness, rash, tiredness, sweating
Ranitidine	Zantac Pylorid	Tablet Effervescent tablet Syrup	150mg, 300mg 150mg, 300mg 75mg/5ml	Gastric and duodenal ulceration: 150mg 2 times/d for 4–8 weeks (max 600mg), maintenance 150mg nocte; prophylaxis of NSAID-induced ulcer 150mg 2 times/d; reflux oesophagitis: 150mg 2 times/d (max 600mg) for up to 12 weeks	Contraindicated in porphyria; caution in hepatic and renal impairment (reduce dose), pregnancy and breast feeding; treatment may mask symptoms of gastric cancer; used to treat dyspepsia due to gastric and duodenal ulceration or NSAID-associated ulceration (also prophylaxis) and reflux oesophagitis	Diarrhoea and other gastrointestinal effects, altered liver function tests, headache, dizziness, rash, tiredness
Ranitidine bismuth citrate (ranitidine bismutrex)		Tablet	400mg	Gastric and duodenal ulceration: 400mg 2 times/d for 4–8 weeks (max 16 weeks treatment/year)	Contraindicated in moderate to severe renal impairment, pregnancy and breast feeding; treatment may mask symptoms of gastric cancer, take after food; used to treat dyspepsia due to gastric and duodenal ulceration; used with clarithromycin and amoxicillin or clarithromycin and metronidazole for *H. pylori* eradication (see also lansoprazole)	Diarrhoea and other gastrointestinal effects, altered liver function tests, headache, dizziness, rash, tiredness; encephalopathy following absorption of bismuth not reported

Drug	Trade name	Preparation	Strength	Doses used in gastrointestinal disease (adult)	Comments	Side-effects
Chelates and complexes						
Tripotassium dicitratobismuthate	De-Noltab	Tablet	120mg	Gastric and duodenal ulceration: 240mg 2 times/d for 4-8 weeks	Contraindicated in renal impairment, pregnancy; treatment may mask symptoms of gastric cancer: used to treat dyspepsia due to gastric and duodenal ulceration: not used alone to maintain remission; take before food	Nausea, vomiting: encephalopathy following absorption of bismuth not reported
Sucralfate	Antepsin	Tablet Suspension	1g 1g/5ml	Gastric and duodenal ulceration: 2g 2 times/d (max 8g/d) for 4-12 weeks	Caution in renal impairment, pregnancy and breast feeding: take before food; used to treat dyspepsia due to gastric and duodenal ulceration	Constipation, diarrhoea, nausea, indigestion, gastric discomfort, dry mouth, rash, hypersensitivity reactions, back pain, dizziness, headache, vertigo, drowsiness
Prostaglandin analogues						
Misoprostol	Cytotec	Tablet	200mcg	Gastric and duodenal ulceration: 400mcg 2 times/d for 4-8 weeks; prophylaxis of NSAID-induced ulcer 200mcg 2 times/d	Contraindicated in pregnancy or planned pregnancy (women of childbearing potential should take effective contraceptive measures); caution in conditions where hypotension may precipitate severe complications (e.g. cerebrovascular and cardiovascular disease); treatment may mask symptoms of gastric cancer: not used alone to maintain remission; take before food	Diarrhoea (may be severe), abdominal pain, flatulence, nausea, vomiting, abnormal vaginal bleeding, rashes, dizziness

Drug	Trade name	Preparation	Strength	Doses used in gastrointestinal disease (adult)	Comments	Side-effects
Proton pump inhibitors						
Esomeprazole	Nexium	Tablet	20mg, 40mg	Gastrointestinal reflux disease: 40mg/d for 4-8 weeks, maintenance 20mg/d	Caution in hepatic and renal impairment (reduce dose), pregnancy, breast feeding; treatment may mask symptoms of gastric cancer; do not take with indigestion mixtures; used with clarithromycin and amoxicillin or metronidazole for H. pylori eradication (see also lansoprazole)	Gastrointestinal effects (diarrhoea, nausea, vomiting, constipation, flatulence, abdominal pain), headache, hypersensitivity reactions (rash, urticaria, angioedema, bronchospasm), pruritus, dizziness, peripheral oedema, muscle and joint pain, malaise, blurred vision, depression, dry mouth
Lansoprazole	Zoton	Capsule	15mg, 30mg	Gastric and duodenal ulceration: 30mg mane for 4-8 weeks, maintenance 15mg mane; prophylaxis of NSAID-induced ulcer: 15-30mg mane for 4-8 weeks; gastrointestinal reflux disease: 30mg mane for 4-8 weeks, maintenance 15-30mg mane	Caution in hepatic impairment (reduce dose), pregnancy, breast feeding; used to treat dyspepsia due to gastric and duodenal ulceration or NSAID-associated ulceration (also prophylaxis) and gastrointestinal reflux disease; treatment may mask symptoms of gastric cancer; do not take with indigestion mixtures	Gastrointestinal effects (diarrhoea, nausea, vomiting, constipation, flatulence, abdominal pain), headache, hypersensitivity reactions (rash, urticaria, angio-oedema, bronchospasm, Stevens-Johnson syndrome, toxic epidermal necrolysis, bullous eruption, erythema multiforme, anaphylaxis), pruritus, dizziness, peripheral oedema, muscle and joint pain, malaise, blurred vision, depression, dry mouth, alopecia, photosensitivity, haematological changes, taste disturbance, vertigo, confusion
		Suspension	30mg/ sachet			

Drug	Trade name	Preparation	Strength	Doses used in gastrointestinal disease (adult)	Comments	Side-effects
Proton pump inhibitors						
Lansoprazole + amoxicillin + clarithromycin	HeliClear	Capsules + tablet	30mg + 500mg + 500mg	H. pylori eradication in patients with duodenal ulcer: 30mg + 500mg + 500mg 2 times/d for 7-14 days	Clarithromycin - caution in renal and hepatic impairment, QT interval prolongation, pregnancy and breast feeding; amoxicillin - contraindicated in penicillin hypersensitivity, caution in allergy; metronidazole - caution in hepatic and renal impairment	Clarithromycin - nausea, vomiting, abdominal discomfort, diarrhoea, urticaria, rashes and other allergic reactions, cardiac effects, headache, smell and taste disturbances, stomatitis, glossitis, dizziness, vertigo, tinnitus, anxiety, insomnia; amoxicillin - nausea, vomiting, diarrhoea, rashes (discontinue treatment); metronidazole - disulfiram-like reaction with alcohol, nausea, vomiting, unpleasant taste, furred tongue, gastrointestinal effects, rashes
Lansoprazole + clarithromycin + metronidazole	HeliMet	Capsule + tablets	30mg + 500mg + 400mg	H. pylori eradication in patients with duodenal ulcer: 30mg + 500mg + 400mg 2 times/d for 7 days		
Omeprazole	Losec	Capsule	10mg, 20mg, 40mg	Gastric and duodenal ulceration, prophylaxis of NSAID-induced ulcer: 20mg/d for 4-8 weeks (max 40mg), maintenance 20mg/d; gastro-intestinal reflux disease: 20mg/d for 4-12 weeks (max 40mg/d), maintenance 20mg/d	Caution in hepatic and renal impairment (reduce dose), pregnancy, breast feeding; used to treat cyspepsia due to gastric and duodenal ulceration and gastro-intestinal reflux disease: treatment may mask symptoms of gastric cancer; do not take with indigestion mixtures; used with clarithromycin and amoxicillin or metronidazole for H. pylori eradication (see also lansoprazole)	Gastrointestinal effects (diarrhoea, nausea, vomiting, constipation, flatulence, abdominal pain), headache, hypersensitivity reactions (rash, urticaria, angio-oedema, bronchospasm, Stevens Johnson syndrome, toxic epidermal necrolysis, bullous eruption, anaphylaxis), fever, alopecia, photosensitivity, somnolence, insomnia, vertigo, sweating
	Losec	Dispersible tablet	10mg, 20mg, 40mg			

Drug	Trade name	Preparation	Strength	Doses used in gastrointestinal disease (adult)	Comments	Side-effects
Proton pump inhibitors						
Pantoprazole	Protium	Capsule	20mg, 40mg	Gastric and duodenal ulceration: 40mg mane for 2-8 weeks; gastrointestinal reflux disease: 40mg mane for 4-8 weeks, maintenance 20mg mane	Caution in hepatic and renal impairment (reduce dose), pregnancy, breast feeding; used to treat dyspepsia due to gastric and duodenal ulceration and gastrointestinal reflux disease; treatment may mask symptoms of gastric cancer; do not take with indigestion mixtures; used with clarithromycin and amoxicillin or metronidazole for *H. pylori* eradication (see also lansoprazole)	Gastrointestinal effects (diarrhoea, nausea, vomiting, constipation, flatulence, abdominal pain), headache, hypersensitivity reactions (rash, urticaria, angio-oedema, bronchospasm, anaphylaxis), pruritus, dizziness, peripheral oedema, muscle and joint pain, malaise, blurred vision, depression, dry mouth, fever, raised triglycerides
Rabeprazole	Pariet	Tablets	10mg, 20mg	Gastric and duodenal ulceration: 20mg mane for 4-12 weeks; gastrointestinal reflux disease: 20mg mane for 4-8 weeks, maintenance 10-20mg mane	Caution in hepatic impairment (reduce dose), pregnancy, breast feeding; used to treat dyspepsia due to gastric and duodenal ulceration and gastrointestinal reflux disease; treatment may mask symptoms of gastric cancer; do not take with indigestion mixtures; used with clarithromycin and amoxicillin or metronidazole for *H. pylori* eradication (see also lansoprazole)	Gastrointestinal effects (diarrhoea, nausea, vomiting, constipation, flatulence, abdominal pain), headache, hypersensitivity reactions (rash, urticaria, angio-oedema, bronchospasm), pruritus, dizziness, peripheral oedema, muscle and joint pain, malaise, blurred vision, depression, dry mouth, stomatitis, chest pain, cough, rhinitis, sinusitis, leucocytosis, insomnia, nervousness, drowsiness, asthenia, taste disturbance, pharyngitis, influenza-like syndrome, sweating, weight gain

Drug	Trade name	Preparation	Strength	Doses used in gastrointestinal disease (adult)	Comments	Side-effects
Gastrointestinal motility stimulants						
Domperidone	Motilium	Tablet	10mg	Functional dyspepsia: 10-20mg 3 times/d and nocte (max 12 weeks)	Caution in pregnancy and breast feeding: used to treat non-ulcer dyspepsia: take before food; not for chronic administration	Raised prolactin concentrations (galactorrhoea and gynaecomastia possible), reduced libido, rashes and other allergic reactions, acute dystonic reactions
		Suspension	10mg/5ml			
Metoclopramide	Maxolon	Tablet	5mg, 10mg	Functional dyspepsia: 10mg (5mg in patients aged 15-19 years <60kg) 3 times/d	Contraindicated in gastrointestinal obstruction, perforation or haemorrhage, for 3-4 days after gastrointestinal surgery. phaeochromocytoma, breast feeding; caution in hepatic and renal impairment (reduce dose), elderly and young adults, pregnancy, po phyria; used to control nausea and vomiting in non-ulcer dyspepsia and gastrointestinal reflux disease	Extrapyramidal effects (especially in young adults), hyperprolactinaemia, tardive dyskinesia (occasionally with prolonged administration), drowsiness, restlessness, diarrhoea, depression, neuroleptic malignant syndrome, rashes, pruritus, oedema
		Syrup	5mg/5ml			
	Maxolon SR	M/R capsule	15mg			
	Gastrobid Continus	M/R tablet	15mg			

Drug	Trade name	Preparation	Strength	Doses used in gastrointestinal disease (adult)	Comments	Side-effects
Gastrointestinal motility stimulants						
Ursodeoxycholic acid	Destolit	Tablet	150mg	Dissolution of gallstones: 8-12mg/kg nocte or in 2 divided doses for 3-4 months after stones dissolve (prophylaxis for up to 2 years)	Contraindicated in radio-opaque stones, pregnancy, non-functioning gall bladder, diseases of the small intestine, colon and liver which interfere with enterohepatic circulation of bile salts; caution in hepatic disease	Nausea, vomiting, diarrhoea, gall stone calcification, pruritus
	Urdox	Tablet	300mg			
	Ursofalk	Capsule	250mg			
		Suspension	250mg/5 ml			

Appendix 2 — Useful Addresses and Websites

Societies

British Society of Gastroenterology
Address: 3 St Andrews Place, Regent's Park, London, NW1 4LB, UK
Tel.: +44 (0) 207 387 3534
Fax: +44 (0) 207 487 3734
Website: http://www.bsg.org.uk/

American College of Gastroenterology
Address: 4900 South 31st Street, Arlington, VA 22206, USA
Tel.: (+1) 703 820 7400
Fax: (+1) 703 931 4520
Website: http://www.acg.gi.org/

American Gastroenterological Association
Address: 7910 Woodmont Avenue, Seventh Floor, Bethesda, MD 20814, USA
Tel.: (+1) 301 654 2055
Fax: (+1) 301 652 3890
Website: http://www.gastro.org/

American Society of Gastrointestinal Endoscopy
Address: 1520 Kensington Road, Suite 202, Oak Brook, IL 60523,USA
Tel.: (+1) 630 573 0600
Fax: (+1) 630 573 0691
Website: http://www.asge.org/

Society of Gastroenterology Nurses & Associates (SGNA)
Address: Secretariat: PO Box 267, Mount Prospect, IL 60056, USA
Tel.: (+1) 847 297 5088
Website: http://www.signea.org/

European Society for Neurogastroenterology & Motility
Website: http://www.neurogastro.org/

Journals

Gastroenterology
Website: http://www2.gastrojournal.org/

Gut
Website: http://gut.bmjjournals.com/

Alimentary Pharmacology & Therapeutics
Website: http://www.blackwell-science.com/products/journals/apt.htm

Digestion (International Journal of Digestion)
Website:
http://content.karger.com/ProdukteDB/produkte.asp?Aktion=JournalHome&ProduktNr=223838&ContentOnly=false

Patient organizations

Digestive Disorders Foundation
Address: The Digestive Disorders Foundation, 3 St Andrew's Place, London, NW1 4L, UK
Tel.: +44 (0) 207 486 0341
Fax: +44 (0) 207 224 2012
Website: http://www.digestivedisorders.org.uk/

International Foundation for Functional Gastroenterological Disorders
Address: PO Box 170864, Milwaukee, WI 53217-8076, USA
Tel.: (+1) 414 964 1799
Fax: (+1) 414 964 7176
Website: http://www.iffgd.org/

The Helicobacter foundation
Website: http://www.helico.com/

Evidence Based Medicine

Centre for Evidence Based Medicine
Website: http://minerva.minervation.com/cebm/

SIGN - Scottish Intercollegiate Guidelines Network
Website: http://www.show.scot.nhs.uk/sign/index.html

Online Databases and Services

GI Diseases Links — Karolinska Institute
Website: http://www.mic.ki.se/Diseases/c6.html

GastroHep
Website: http://www.gastrohep.com/

Index

Notes:

As the subject of this book is dyspepsia, entries under this term have been kept to a minimum: readers are advised to seek more specific entries. This index is presented in letter-by-letter order, whereby spaces and hyphens in main entries are excluded from the alphabetization process. Page numbers followed by the letters 'f' and 't' refer to figures and tables respectively.